Bikini Bootcamp

Bikini Bootcamp

Two Weeks to Your
Ultimate Beach Body

MELISSA PERLMAN AND ERICA GRAGG

ILLUSTRATIONS BY DIANA MARYE HUFF

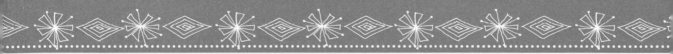

BROADWAY BOOKS | NEW YORK

BROADWAY

Published by Broadway Books

Copyright © 2007 by Amansala USA, LLC, and Peele
Enterprises, LLC

Published in the United States by Broadway Books, an im-
print of The Doubleday Broadway Publishing Group, a di-
vision of Random House, Inc., New York.
www.broadwaybooks.com

Broadway Books and its logo, a letter B bisected on the
diagonal, are trademarks of Random House, Inc.

Book design by Nancy Campana
Illustrations by Diana Marye Huff

Library of Congress Cataloging-in-Publication Data

Perlman, Melissa, 1965–
Bikini bootcamp : Two weeks to your ultimate beach body /
Melissa Perlman and Erica Gragg; illustrations by Diana
Marye Huff.—1st ed.
p.   cm.
ISBN 978-0-7679-2590-7
1. Women—Health and hygiene—Popular works. 2.
Women—Nutrition—Popular works. 3. Reducing diets—
Popular works.
4. Self-care, Health. I. Gragg, Erica. II. Title.
RA778.P34 2007
613.7—dc22
2006037776

Printed in the United States of America

1   3   5   7   9   10   8   6   4   2

First Edition

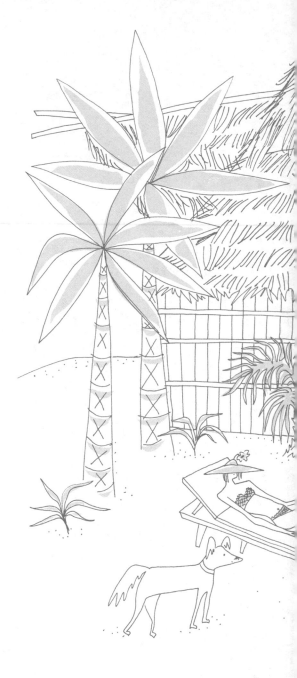

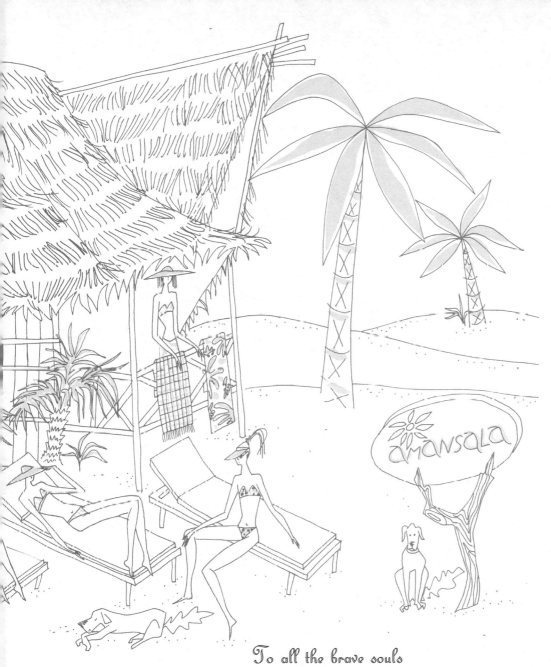

To all the brave souls
who came to Bikini Bootcamp and encouraged us along the way.

And to our wonderful staff,
who have become our family here on the beach in Mexico.

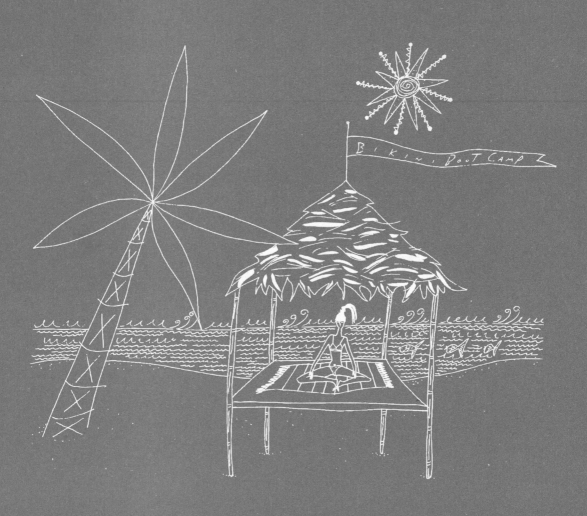

contents

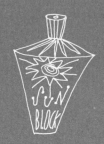

Welcome to Bikini Bootcamp

The best way to make your dreams come true is to wake up.
—*Anonymous*

Like many great stories, Bikini Bootcamp started with a simple idea: to sublet our apartments; pack a few bags with beach clothes; gather some nice sheets, linens, incense, and candles; and host weekend getaways for busy city dwellers like ourselves on a glorious stretch of unspoiled beach on the Mexican Riviera. We'd name our imaginary hotel Amansala, Sanskrit for "peaceful place on the water." Our philosophy would be simple: "back to basics with style and comfort," a place where guests could come to reconnect to themselves and nature through healthy eating, a variety of activities like yoga, kayaking, workouts on the beach, and, of course, a bit of pampering.

At first we focused on folks like us—urban workaholics who could get away only for weekend jaunts. But then we realized that there was actually a huge demand for more extended vacations with a purpose—time away from daily pressures that rejuvenates the body and mind through an experience that challenges you and helps you grow. So we created an actual program and called it Bikini Bootcamp.

Little did we know that this simple idea would quickly turn into a journey that would transform our lives—and the lives of the thousands of visitors who participate in our program each year. In the four years since its inception, Bikini Bootcamp has grown from a fantasy into a proven program for weight loss, body transformation, and spiritual growth.

The two of us had been best friends for years, experiencing the best and worst of New York City as single career women with busy lives and endless adventures. Melissa had traveled, lived, and worked all over the world, spending many years as a student of Buddhism and meditation while she lived and journeyed in the Far East, and stayed at all sorts of resorts from the most deluxe to the most rustic. She had been toying with the idea of creating an ecologically friendly yet stylish retreat, where visitors could renew themselves and escape from the stress of modern life. It would be a place where guests could eat healthy and improve their bodies and minds in a way that would last long after their suntan faded. Meanwhile, Erica had recently become a fitness and yoga instructor; she had a great job in public relations but was looking to bring more purpose into her life.

After 9/11, that need became all the more clear. Some of our friends lost loved ones; others lost jobs. Melissa worked as a volunteer near Ground Zero, and Erica went to church, this time praying for something more than a really hot date. The tragedy of 9/11 and the quantum shift in society that followed made the need to enjoy the simple things and bring more spiritual meaning into everyone's lives a priority.

To develop the Bikini Bootcamp program, we studied virtually every hot diet out there—from Atkins to Sugar Busters to eating according to your blood type. We consulted with registered nutritionists and top chefs. Through trial and error, we realized that most of the popular diets on the market can confuse your metabolism and make it very difficult to shed pounds or even maintain a healthy weight. We also learned that losing weight and staying healthy, trim, and fit is actually much simpler than anybody seems to realize—or wants to admit. The secret to slimming down and maintaining a bikini-ready body for a lifetime is to eat nutritious, low-fat, and fiber-packed foods that are as close to their natural form as possible. After all, we don't have to count calories to know that a salad is a better choice than french fries. As a trained chef who had once run her own restaurant in Japan, Melissa was able to devise sumptuous dishes, a fusion of Mexican and Asian cuisines, that reflect our philosophy and get results.

To develop our body-shaping programs we also sought the advice of professionals in the fields of exercise, body mechanics, yoga, and meditation. Erica had studied every fitness method under the sun—from stripper workouts to Pilates and everything in between—so she was able to bring to the mix a personal knowledge of what really works and what's actually doable for busy women. The result is an uncomplicated, workable, and balanced fitness, eating, and living plan that evolved into the Bikini Bootcamp Lifestyle. All that remained was to put our plan into action.

Needless to say, finding the perfect location for our boot camp was a priority. We knew our dream resort had to be located in Tulum, on Mexico's Caribbean coast. Melissa had been introduced to this uniquely beautiful and isolated ten-kilometer stretch of white sand beach bordered by a calm, clear, turquoise sea ten years earlier, and it had drawn her back many times. Unlike other formerly idyllic vacation spots around the Caribbean, Tulum's peace and tranquility have remained untouched, thanks to unpaved access roads, no big hotels, and the often unpredictable availability of water, lights, and plumbing. So the sun still beams down on water that is crystalline pure, and the starry nightscape is as wondrous today as it was thousands of years ago. All this made Tulum the ideal spot for what we thought of as an "eco-chic fitness retreat." Plus, the beach was close to several stunning sites that we could incorporate into our guests' experience; the gleaming white ruins of Tulum's pre-Hispanic Mayan city were less than an hour away by bike, and the Cenote Tankah—a system of freshwater pools made of natural limestone and coral wells that lead to underground rivers, caverns, and cave systems—would make for great snorkeling excursions for our visitors.

We decided to take a leap of faith and set about putting our plan into action. We built a website describing the resort we *hoped* we'd build, and the kind of fitness program we *hoped* to create. We sent out information to a variety of magazines who eagerly wrote about a new fitness getaway called Bikini Bootcamp, and to our amazement, people started signing up! The only problem was that, at this point, Bikini Bootcamp existed only in our minds. Oops! We told all of our would-be guests that we were booked for six months and decided we'd better get on a plane to Mexico and get busy . . . Of course, the "no vacancies" excuse piqued our guests' interest even more.

When we arrived in Mexico, we lugged our six enormous duffel bags down to a small beach town with no electricity, no running water, and no real infrastructure. We spent our first night in a sandy-floored room at a hotel catering to backpackers, sharing with the other guests a dark, out-door bathroom that seemed to be crawling with creepy creatures.

We hitched rides down dusty roads in the back of anything with wheels—a wobbly old truck filled with bananas, and even a shiny new po-lice car, the nicest ride in town. We found a variety of run-down cabanas, but they were too grungy to fit our vision. Just as we were about to give up, we saw a cluster of thatched-roofed cabanas nestled among lazily wav-ing palm trees. Even better, we heard the sound of a hammer. Melissa found the owner, a Mayan local flashing gold front teeth, making repairs. He showed us the property. Yes, it was a mess—no electricity or running water—but it had potential. A few weeks later we were the proud new owners of Rancho Amansala.

We moved our duffels into one of the unfinished cabanas. Electricians, carpenters, and plumbers, all claiming to be experts, appeared out of the jungle after word spread that the crazy *Americanas* were hiring. Melissa took control of the crew and, with her broken Spanish, became the fore-man. Before this, the closest she had gotten to managing a construction crew was calling her building's superintendent to come to her apartment and hang a picture!

Slowly, Amansala began to take shape. Natural stone floors replaced the sand, and proper beds arrived. We draped romantic (and practical) mosquito nets over them, decorated the bathrooms with local mosaics, and

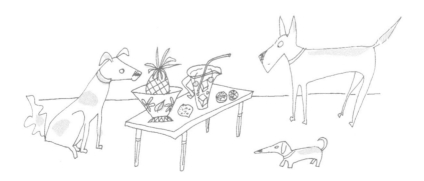

painted the walls tropical shades of pink, yellow, and orange. It quickly began to look like Bikini Bootcamp was on its way to becoming a reality.

Naturally, when we first opened in November 2002, everything that could go wrong did. Employees didn't show up, pipes broke, the chef drank, tropical storms rolled in. But slowly, we learned how to run a resort and our community started to take shape: local fishermen, the hardworking staff, curious locals, stray beach dogs that wandered up to the hotel and became beloved four-legged friends, and, of course, a variety of guests.

We quickly got over our growing pains, and Bikini Bootcamp at Amansala soon became a sensation as a fitness destination and yoga retreat center. With no advertising, Bikini Bootcamp now hosts over three thousand guests each year and is booked several months in advance thanks to word-of-mouth recommendations from satisfied customers. To our delight, it's become *the* place for urban hipsters, socialites, and celebrities as well as thousands of people simply in search of a trimmer figure and a bit more meaning in their lives. A visit to Bikini Bootcamp is a back-to-basics tune-up for the mind, body, and spirit, away from the hectic pace of daily life. At Amansala, the electricity shuts off at ten, there's no need for hair-dryers and BlackBerries, and food is really a simple pleasure, made with fresh, local ingredients. But we also provide Bikini Bootcamp spa treatments *à la Mexicano* to rejuvenate our guests after a long day. Our guests can enjoy a massage in the afternoon or slather their bodies with local clays reputed to heal anything that ails you and to firm and tone the skin. They can also try our papaya and avocado facials—easy beauty rituals guaranteed to make your complexion shine.

We have traded our Gucci stilettos for flip-flops, but the changes reach far beyond our wardrobe. We have learned more than we ever thought possible about how to take care of ourselves and our guests, body and soul. Our guests range from housewives to high-powered executives, to recent college grads, to mothers and daughters. Away from their cell phones, computers, families, work, and all other responsibilities, our guests are able to focus on nurturing themselves. Many arrive exhausted and stressed, but they all leave replenished, having been pampered from the inside out, with a new blueprint for eating well and maintaining their new physique.

It follows, then, that Bikini Bootcamp is not just another exercise/eat right/how-to book. This book brings to you, dear readers, our own unique take on getting healthy and in shape. Normally, the words "boot camp" conjure up the image of a drill sergeant barking orders in your face for another fifty push-ups as sweat rolls down your neck, your muscles burn in protest, and you silently wonder, "Won't this ever end?" That kind of boot camp harkens back to the tired and ultimately unsuccessful fitness cliché, "no pain, no gain." That kind of workout might leave you gasping for breath with marginally tighter abs—but it's also impossible to tolerate for long. The traditional boot camp is designed to shock the system; it's not intended to be a program you can do for life. Furthermore, we know that realistically it's not possible to re-create that kind of atmosphere at home. And who would really want to?

So we've combined the concept of boot camp (tough stuff) with a more practical, feminine (bikini) approach. Think of our Bikini Bootcamp as a softer approach to harder bodies. Our method works—not only does it give you results as quickly as any sergeant's workout, but it also provides maintainable results that will last much longer. And, best of all, it makes your body and mind feel *good*.

While you may not be able to take your morning walks on a secluded cove of sand, followed by a refreshing dip in the Caribbean Sea, or use fresh-picked coconuts for weights during your circuit training regimen, you can easily incorporate the Bikini Bootcamp program into your daily life no matter where you are. Without ever going to Mexico, you, too, can give yourself the same kick-start to a healthier, leaner body by following the step-by-step body, lifestyle, and nutritional program that's laid out clearly for you in Part II of this book.

Just like Bikini Bootcamp guests who revel in the beauty of Tulum's fabled beach, we'll show you how to find beauty and inspiration in your own environment and rediscover the fun and joy that comes with moving your body and quieting your mind. You'll dine on delicious, slenderizing dishes that evoke the exotic flavors of the Mayan Riviera and enjoy simple yet luxurious do-it-yourself spa treatments—exactly what we offer our guests and using the same all-natural ingredients that are found in many brand-name beauty products. And at the end of two weeks, you'll be able to slip into that bikini feeling stronger, slimmer, and more confident, and knowing you have that inner glow that comes from feeling healthy, balanced, and restored. You'll be able to hit the beach wherever you are.

The Bikini Bootcamp program combines aerobic exercise (in the form of walking), circuit training, our specially designed core abs and back series, and yoga into a uniquely simple and time-effective daily routine that takes the guesswork out of fitness—and reshapes your body. Our exercises will make you more conscious and aware of your movements and physique—maybe even for the first time. And by blending yoga with cardio and core-strengthening exercises, all designed to elongate, tone, and strengthen your muscles, your circulation and posture will also improve.

Although most people come to Amansala to shape up or jump-start a fitness regimen, the changes go far beyond attaining a smaller dress size. Week after week, we see guests transform their bodies, reshape thighs, flatten tummies, clear their skin, and regain a sparkle in their eyes.

Now, after nearly four years of diligently perfecting the Bikini Bootcamp program, this book gives our guests—and you—the one thing you all crave: a way to take our program home, transforming a one-week stay into a fourteen-day health and fitness makeover that will give you a bikini body for a lifetime.

Believe it or not, you *can* lose up to ten pounds and tone those winter thighs in just two weeks, so you can feel good about yourself and be full of energy just in time for beach season—or any season at all. One repeat Bikini Bootcamper, Samantha, has lost a grand total of forty-five pounds by taking the program home with her. Over the next fourteen days, you can expect to lose between four to ten pounds, depending on your current weight and fitness level. But this is only the beginning. The Bikini Bootcamp Program is a kick-start to your Bikini Bootcamp Lifestyle, guaranteed to help you reach your ideal shape and stay healthy, energized, and fit for years to come.

....

Did you know that in just two weeks, you can build a pound of muscle? You will also increase your metabolic rate and burn 30 to 50 more calories a day. That's 210 to 350 extra calories burned per week!

....

Our program is user-friendly and practical—perfect for anyone who has trouble finding the time to keep fit. Bikini Bootcamp workouts are designed to be broken down into short, convenient blocks of time during the day, with no fancy equipment, no gym membership, and no personal trainers needed. Ever.

Even better, our concept encourages compliance—and *everyone* knows all too well that the primary reason most fitness/diet programs fail is due to noncompliance. Programs and diets tend either to be too tough, complicated, time-consuming, boring, or too dependent on expensive gym sessions and classes. Furthermore, it's been proven time and again that dieting alone does not work. Nutritional programs can and do work, but they must be combined with the right type of regular exercise plan or you set yourself up for failure. The wrong program will discourage you and derail your focus; soon you'll begin to believe that you can't really change and might as well stick with the status quo. If that's been your experience in the past, Bikini Bootcamp is the solution. It's fun, it's easy, and it gets fast results.

The Bikini Bootcamp eating plan is high in fiber, lean proteins, healthy fats, and healthy carbs. We don't count calories—after all, this isn't about dieting, but establishing lifelong eating habits in which you give your body only quality fuel. Quality fuel does not mean deprivation. As you will see when you start following the recipes in Part III, good eating means delicious eating. Our food is ultrasimple, made with fresh local ingredients. These days, farmers' markets, organic food markets, and even local supermarkets are getting on the fresh food bandwagon, making it easy for you to duplicate our recipes at home. Our guests savor meals packed with tropical fruits, ripe vegetables, healthy proteins like fish and chicken, and whole grains that are free of processed fats and flavoring, and so will you. Getting back to basics is the most effective way to give your body what it needs to be healthy, slim down, and feel great. In fact, getting back to basics means eating the way that our ancestors naturally ate—fresh fruits, veggies, and lean meats and fish—before the assembly-line approach to food production processed and refined the nutrition out of our foods, and then added chemicals to boot.

So, if you're worried about having to give up your fast-food habit or that coffee with a donut-bagel-muffin breakfast you're addicted to, don't worry. Your taste in food will quickly change when you start eating the Bikini Bootcamp way, so that you will no longer crave heavily sugared, re-fined, or fatty foods full of chemical additives. Our guests are amazed to return home and find themselves reaching for fruit instead of cookies, or crisp green salad instead of pasta. This is why you will never have to diet; because your new healthy eating habits will ensure that your weight won't creep back up and that your energy stays consistent and strong.

Over the next two weeks we'll also introduce you to the Bikini Body Mind-set, which will release you from self-made traps that keep you stuck in old habits, and free you to set brand-new fitness goals. By now we've all heard about how meditation can do wonders for your mind and body, and it often seems like everyone today is a practitioner—from the Dalai Lama to Madonna. So what's the deal with meditation, really, and how can it help you with your Bikini Bootcamp transformation? Well, our easy, ten-minute meditations will put you in the right frame of mind to accomplish whatever challenges come your way, including staying focused on the program—even when you're tired or tempted to slip.

Meditation teaches you how to take each day moment by moment, one step at a time, and stay focused on the present, without worrying about how you will do in the future or the unhealthy choices you've made in the past. It increases your awareness of the world around you both emotionally and physically—from the food you eat to the way your body feels and what it really needs. It teaches you how to distinguish true hunger from eating out of habit or emotional need, and it helps calm you whenever you become stressed out, so that rather than running to the nearest vending machine or fridge for a sugary, fat-laden, pound-packing fix, you can take a few moments for meditative breathing—anytime, anywhere—and feel those impulses subside.

If you've never tried meditation, or feel like it's boring or just too New Age for you, we encourage you to give it a try. Even our most skeptical guests—the ones who come prepared to simply eat as little and work out as hard as possible—find that they really benefit from this component of the program. One Bikini Bootcamper, a woman named Susan, told us, "Bikini Bootcamp was a great place for me to reexamine my diet, my exercise routines, and learn simple meditation techniques that I can do anywhere to bring balance and reduce stress. It's made a big difference in how my family eats and relates to each other as a whole."

We also invite you to hone your Bikini Body Mind-set through journaling. How does journaling help you get the body you want? By helping you own your thoughts and feelings and set concrete goals to guide you through the next two weeks. When you journal, you allow whatever comes into your mind to flow out onto paper, without criticism or judgment. This way, you are never able to lie to yourself about your true fears, emotions, or desires. Once you write them down on paper, you actually feel relieved and are less likely to try holding your feelings inside by stuffing them down with food, especially the wrong foods. Putting your goals down on paper also makes them feel more real—and you will be more likely to remain committed to the process if you can open your journal for a reminder every day.

Many of us have a natural tendency to think that we need to make a million changes in our lives overnight. Yet the more we feel we need to do, the more paralyzed or discouraged we can become. Bikini Bootcamp will change the course of your life and the shape of your body one step at a time—but you'll see that these little steps add up quickly. Another guest, Lisa, wrote us a month after she returned home: "You would be proud to know I have made subtle changes in my life that are taking hold. Instead of going to the office at six a.m., I have been walking/running along the Chicago lakefront every morning and writing in my journal daily. I have stopped skipping breakfast and drink my favorite Bikini Bootcamp Smoothie religiously before work so I am no longer starving at lunch. All this has made it possible for me to cut out refined flour and sugar and be much more deliberate about what I eat. I feel great and I'm happy with my body. I can't believe how easy it's been for me to make these changes, and what big results have come from the seeds you planted at BBC."

You'll learn the same lessons and take similar life-altering steps by following the road map laid out in these pages. Even our fitness program is designed to do more than tone your body—it also trains your mind. The stronger you are physically, the better you can cope with all the little obstacles life throws your way—be it an unexpected deadline or a sudden crisis (living on the coast of Mexico, where hurricanes are known to ravage the shoreline, we know a thing or two about that!). Plus, your increased self-awareness and focus will have an enormous impact on your general attitude, creating a more positive outlook that will keep you slim, toned, and healthy for a lifetime.

Finally, the spa experiences included in the book—do-it-yourself beauty treatments made with all-natural ingredients—will give you the gorgeous, glowing, taut skin that everyone wants and remind you of how important it is to take brief respites from your day—even if they're only for ten minutes—so you can relax, unwind, and renew. These spa treats also reinforce our message that Bikini Bootcamp is ultimately about taking care of yourself, and that you are worthy of this level of care always.

Everyone knows that all work and no play makes life a chore rather than a pleasure. Part of the Bikini Bootcamp Mind-set is remembering to have *fun!* Our guests enjoy so much about the Bikini Bootcamp experience besides the workouts and the delicious, healthy food—from sleeping in our thatch-roofed cabanas to swinging in hammocks under palm trees to waking up as the birds greet the sunrise. Our morning beach walks are led by our BBC dogs—Sol, Luna, Pablito, and Azul—who delight our guests with their wagging tails and immediate acceptance and affection. A stay at Bikini Bootcamp would not be the same without these furry friends, and guests are always asking if they can take one of our "friends" home! And although most of our guests arrive alone—and stressed!—no one goes through Bikini Bootcamp by themselves. They sit down to their meals at communal tables, they make friends, support each other along the way, and always exchange contact information to keep up with each other's progress. We will show you how to include experiences like these in your program that will make your two weeks of at-home Bikini Bootcamp just as memorable and pleasurable.

When our guests first arrive at Bikini Bootcamp, we ask them to look at each day as either an opportunity to stay where they are . . . or to view each day as a first step toward where they truly want to be. And then we pose the following questions:

- Do you feel comfortable in your body?
- Can you envision yourself feeling better about yourself?
- How do you feel after a workout?
- What physical activities do you enjoy (such as walking, jogging, yoga, dancing)?
- How do you feel after you eat specific foods?
- Are you happy with where you are in your life?
- What do you plan to achieve by being here with us this week? What is your intention?

By honestly answering these questions, guests are able to pinpoint their specific goals, get focused, and begin working toward the ultimate goal: living in balance with a fit, healthy body, nourished by good food, good fun, good work, and good company.

Now we're asking you to choose. You can look at each day as either an opportunity to stay where you are . . . or view each day as another first step in the direction of where you truly want to be. Ask yourself the same questions we pose to our guests before they commit to Bikini Bootcamp. This way, you can assess your hopes and aspirations, sharpen your focus, and begin creating a fit, healthy, balanced life for yourself.

So let's get ready to hit the beach!

The BBC Credo

We believe . . .

- the key to a healthy, fit body starts with the mind.
- in having fun while working out.
- in taking a proactive approach to health and fitness.
- that exercise and eating well should never be boring, time-consuming, unrealistic, or a chore.
- the thought of working out should not inspire dread.
- that results come from consistency—you should never be able to mess up a program with one or two little slips.
- that the Bikini Bootcamp program will work for you—no matter what your goals.

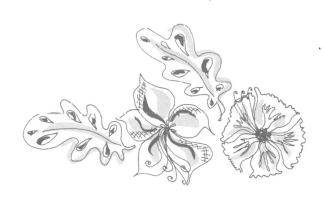

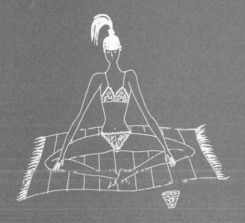

PART I

The Basics

If one advances confidently in the direction of his dreams,
and endeavors to live the life which he has imagined, he will
meet with success in unexpected and uncommon hours.
—Henry David Thoreau

Bikini Bootcamp (BBC) is more than a ticket to a bikini-ready body in just two weeks. It is the start of a brand-new life, in which healthy living becomes a top priority and in which you *consistently* move your body and become conscious about how you nourish yourself, not only with food and drink, but also with the power of positive intention and daily inspiration. It will help you find a new pace of life, one that brings you back to feeling good both physically and mentally, and will leave you feeling refreshed and restored, even if you're working out harder than you have in a long time.

Keep in mind that the BBC program is not work or penance for getting out of shape. We think of BBC less as a workout and more as a way to put play into your day, because our primary aim with our workouts is to restore your childlike joy in movement. Physical motion is a necessity of life. Remember how great it felt to exercise your body as a kid? As you skipped rope and played tag for hours, you weren't thinking about your fitness level or body shape—you were thinking "fun." At Bikini Bootcamp in Mexico, the sun, sand, sea, and camaraderie remind campers of the joy they once had in their bodies, so that improving and maintaining fitness and seeing the pounds disappear is transformed from a sweating, grunting, groaning obligation to pure pleasure.

Regular Exercise Banishes the Blues

Why exactly does BBC leave you both fit and smiling? It's due to an increased release of feel-good hormones called endorphins. A study of depressed adults, published in *Preventive Medicine,* found that mental benefits of a twelve-week training program remained significant when measured twelve months later. Plus, the exposure to sunlight you get during outdoor exercise is particularly helpful during winter's dark months, when your body produces more melatonin, which some researchers believe can cause symptoms of depression. Another reason to seek sunshine wherever you are!

As you go through your own Bikini Bootcamp, you'll learn exercises that tone, strengthen, stretch, and align your body. Our program is not for sissies, but there's no drill sergeant barking commands, either. Instead, you will discover your own inner general by figuring out what's best for *your* individual body. You will start slow to build up stamina gradually and allow you to relish each positive change in your energy level and fitness. You'll learn how to prepare our much-loved Amansala recipes on your own—delicious meals that will nourish you and help you shed weight and add muscle without ever feeling deprived. And our daily meditations and journaling exercises will help you get to the root of any negative eating habits. Knowledge is power, and when you know which foods, people, or situations cause you to make unhealthy eating choices, you can use this awareness to stay on track. We guarantee that no matter what your current shape, size, or fitness level, if you practice this simple, fun, practical program consistently and adopt the Bikini Bootcamp Lifestyle, you will get remarkable results—from the inside out. Looking good for beach season then becomes an option all year round!

The Four Fitness Components of Bikini Bootcamp

At Bikini Bootcamp, our fitness regimen is built around four types of workouts:

1. **Circuit Training** (weight training for specific muscles): 40 minutes every day.
2. **Core Strengthening** (works your back, gluteal muscles, and abdominals): 20 minutes, every other day.
3. **Yoga** (promotes cardiovascular fitness/strength/toning/elongating/destressing): 15 minutes every day.
4. **Walking** (promotes cardiovascular fitness/aerobic capacity/destressing): one hour every day.

Each kind of workout is crucial to getting the results you want, and together they encompass the five types of exercise that lead to a firm and healthy body:

Strength: Our workouts increase muscular and functional strength, which leads to more efficient calorie burning and reshapes and tones your muscles.

Cardio: Cardiovascular exercise strengthens and protects the heart and lungs, increasing your aerobic endurance and power, burning calories, and improving your mood thanks to increased levels of feel-good endorphins.

Flexibility: Our workouts are designed to help you increase the range of motion in your joints and develop greater muscle suppleness and ease of movement. Stretching lengthens your muscles for a flattering long and slender—rather than bulked-up—look.

Core: Engaging the deep muscles of your core, or torso, improves your overall stability, coordination, balance, strength, and prevents back injury and aches. Plus, it's the key to having a slim, taut, and sexy tummy.

Restorative: Our stretches, found at the end of our circuit training and yoga sequences, relieve physical and mental stress, beat the blues, increase energy, and improve your alignment, coordination, balance, and stability.

It's Not Just about the Bikini

Remember that the benefits of exercise go far beyond having a bathing suit body. Studies show that regular exercise reduces the risk of high blood pressure and heart disease by up to 50 percent. A study published in the *Journal of Clinical Epidemiology* found that women between ages 55 and 69 who exercise regularly cut their risk of developing noninsulin-dependent diabetes in half. And according to the American Institute for Cancer Research, women who exercise regularly are 30 to 40 percent less likely to develop breast cancer. You'll also be glad to know that a survey of 408 students at the University of Arkansas found that 88 percent of the women and 69 percent of the men who worked out four to five days a week rated their sexual performance average or way above average, and that they perceived themselves as being more confident and sexually desirable. What could be better than that?

If you're not familiar with any of these kinds of exercises, don't worry! Every activity listed will be explained through clear illustrations and easy-to-follow instructions. We've removed all the guesswork and laid out everything for you in a simple, day-by-day guide. At Bikini Bootcamp we take life the Mexican way—one day at a time. Each day's activities are posted on a large chalkboard the night before, so that our Bikini Bootcampers don't have to make decisions about what they should or shouldn't do; we've found that our guests are tired of having to make choices and actually enjoy being told what to do, where to be, and, especially relating to food, what to eat. How many times have you had a conversation about where or what kind of food to eat? Our program frees you from all that. Our back-to-basics food is delicious and easy to prepare, and we've laid out the meal plans with clear and detailed recipes and other instructions so that you'll feel as if we're your own personal coaches, right there with you every step of the way!

Bikini Bootcamp grads tell us that once they become hooked on moving their bodies regularly, the benefits add up quickly. But we know that gearing up to start or even return to a routine can be tough. So BBC is also designed to give you the motivation and instruction you need to get over that first hurdle and keep moving and smiling. After all, it's the enjoyment you get from regularly moving and challenging your body that will ensure that you maintain your remarkable results. So now let's take a closer look at each of the four workouts and how they will help you get ready for the beach.

Bikini Tip: A Lack of Free Time Is No Excuse!

Our workouts are designed to be broken down into shorter intervals if necessary, so no matter how busy or overextended you are, you'll be able to squeeze in time for the program here and there. You're guaranteed to feel great after a day or two, and that will motivate you to find time to do more. We hope that the changes you see will inspire you to take charge of your schedule, instead of letting it take charge of you.

CHAPTER 1

Circuit Training

One's destination is never a place but rather a new way of looking at things.
—*Henry Miller*

Circuit training is the easiest way to incorporate a full-body workout into your busy schedule, and you don't even have to go to the gym! Simply put, circuit training alternates brief intervals of strength-training exercises, like push-ups, with bursts of cardiovascular activity, like jumping rope. It's one of the best and most efficient ways to fire up your metabolism and sculpt and tone your muscles, head to toe.

Many of you may already work out regularly—running outdoors or on a treadmill, cycling on an exercise bike, or taking aerobics classes. But it's not enough to continue the same workout, month after month. When our muscles become accustomed to doing specific exercises, they are no longer challenged. It's not that exercising becomes a waste of time, because any sustained aerobic exercise is good for the cardiovascular system, but it will no longer be as effective at improving muscle tone or burning calories.

Sticking to the same workout also makes it easy for us to grow complacent, even lazy, once we hit that plateau where nothing seems to happen. In fact, those people you see in the gym reading magazines while slowly pedaling on the exercise bike can even wind up *gaining* weight. You don't want to be one of them! Physiologically, the human body is designed to respond to a challenge. That's where circuit training comes in.

Circuit training alternates strength and cardio exercises performed in quick succession so you're forced to focus on the task at hand and your body naturally follows. It's impossible to do a BBC cardio circuit while watching TV or talking to your friend on a cell phone. The constantly changing exercises challenge your attention and concentration—and when you focus on following the routine exactly, you cannot cheat or become complacent. Furthermore, the muscle you build through circuit training raises your body's metabolic rate, so you burn more calories even when you are at rest, and that translates into dropping pounds and staying slim. You will find that your functional mobility, strength, and stamina all improve dramatically with our three BBC circuit training routines. You'll lose inches, tone your body, look better, feel better, and add challenge and variety to your workout. If your usual cardio routine has been putting you to sleep, BBC circuit training is the solution because it blasts you out of your fitness rut!

Circuit training is very easy to fit into your life. Just make a commitment to move, and, before you know it, you'll be getting results. You can circuit train in a gym, if that's what you prefer, but you won't need an expensive gym membership, special equipment, or workout clothes to do the circuits we've outlined here. With just a little creativity, circuit training can be done anywhere—in your home, a hotel room, a park, or even in your office cubicle during lunch hour. Don't have hand weights? Try soup cans, water bottles, rocks, or books instead. At BBC in Mexico, we actually use coconuts that we pick from our own trees (they're heavier than you might think!). So, you can purchase some coconuts from your local supermarket if you want to add a little atmosphere. We advise that you work the circuit at whatever level challenges you, increasing the intensity and duration of the exercises as your fitness level soars. And because there are so many great exercises to choose from, we've mixed and matched in order to vary your circuit training workout from day to day. Variety is half the fun—and, as we've seen, the key to dramatic and lasting body changes.

Bikini Bootcamp circuits consist of a series of strength exercises, completed one after another in fairly quick succession, with two-minute bursts of cardio spaced in between each series to keep your heart rate high. Each strength exercise is performed for one minute, so that the muscle being worked reaches fatigue before you move on to the next exercise. Each exercise is also separated by a fifteen-second interval, to give you a chance to grab your new equipment and change position.

Bikini Tip: Stay Hydrated

At Bikini Bootcamp we chant the mantra, Water, Water Water! And not just because we're on the beach all day. No matter the season or the locale, you want to keep your energy high by drinking at least four to six 8-ounce glasses of water a day. During your Bikini Bootcamp program, boost your intake to eight glasses.

The great thing about doing BBC circuits is that you never have to count reps. All you do is watch the clock and move on to the next exercise when your minute is up. Bear in mind, however, that you should never sacrifice quality of form for speed. The BBC philosophy holds that fewer reps accomplished well and with maximum concentration are better than a high number of poorly executed reps. Good form is also crucial to avoid injury and for any exercise to accomplish its intended results, so follow our directions closely. After a while, you will find that your body adjusts to each exercise, and as you develop more strength and stamina, you will naturally increase the number of reps in your one-minute period.

What You'll Need

- A mat
- Light weights *or* coconuts, large soup cans, one-liter water bottles, rocks, or books (three pounds each if you're out of shape, five pounds if you've been exercising regularly)
- Jump rope
- A towel
- Cross trainers or aerobic shoes
- Music that makes you want to move!

A sturdy jump rope costs less than twenty dollars. It can be woven of natural fiber or plastic, and the handles can be either plastic or wood. If you're a beginner, plastic ropes are better because they are easier to swing and unlikely to tangle. Avoid weighted ropes and speed ropes that spin extra quickly, unless you're already a jumping pro. To make sure your rope is the right size for you, step on the middle; the handles should reach to just below your armpits.

If you don't have all these items, don't worry. You can use a towel for your mat, and when it comes time to do your cardio, simply pretend to jump rope, as we often do at Amansala. Just imagine a rope in your hands and visualize it as you jump. Or, substitute jumping jacks instead. Don't forgo the proper shoes, though, as you want to make sure your feet are stable and provide cushioning and support for your ankles and knees.

You should have your equipment close at hand and ready to go prior to starting your workout. If you have the space, create "stations" for each exercise that form a circle; you can even write the name of an exercise on a piece of paper to remind yourself what to do when you get there. Once you complete all the exercises at each station in the circle, you have logged a single circuit.

What's in Your Workout

Circuit training enables you to quickly and easily perform a variety of different types of exercises, all of which have different benefits. You'll be targeting each of your body's distinct muscle groups for a total body-sculpting effect.

Cardio

The cardio component of circuit training is designed to elevate your heart rate in short bursts throughout the workout. For BBC cardio you will jump rope (or simulate jumping rope) or, if you cannot jump because of back or knee problems, march in place with high knees. Cardio exercises also provide an endorphin rush that relieves stress and boosts energy.

You should always choose a jumping spot with "give," like grass, sand, carpeting (but avoid heavy pile), a yoga mat, or a wooden floor. No matter how old you are, you will discover that jumping rope is a fun and effective cardio exercise. What better way to shake off the cares of our busy lives and feel like a kid again?

If you choose to circuit train in a gym, be sure to mix up the cardio machines, alternating between steppers, the elliptical trainer, step aerobics, an inclined treadmill, or ski track.

Lower Body Toners

These exercises will work your leg and gluteal muscles (otherwise known as the glutes or buttocks), and, in most cases, the core muscles as well.

Upper Body Toners

We women tend to focus on typical problem areas like our abdomens, butts, and thighs, but the upper body is equally important to creating your bikini look. A strong, toned upper body and arms will keep you graceful, aligned, and balanced, and shapely shoulders help you look great in bathing suits, tank tops, strapless dresses, and other sexy summer wear.

Plus, working your upper body (and, in particular, your pecs) can give you a lift in all the right areas and ensure that your bust is perky rather than saggy. These exercises will also correct rounded shoulders and encourage you to stand tall, poised, and elegant wherever you are—whether you're commanding the boardroom or on the beach.

Abdominal Toners
A strong, toned abdomen is the centerpiece of the Bikini Bootcamp body, and these exercises will give you the taut tummy you want while at the same time strengthening your back and improving your posture. Each circuit routine includes a special three-minute series of abs that you do at the very end before your cooldown and stretch. Some of these terrific, super-slimming exercises will be used in your core strength routines as well.

Bikini Tip

According to a study conducted at the University of Nebraska at Omaha, pulling your belly button toward the floor during twist crunches (as in Circuit B) makes your oblique muscles work up to 50 percent harder.

The Circuit

In this book we've provided you with three circuit-training courses: Circuit A, Circuit B, and Circuit C—enough variety to keep you from getting bored but not so much that you'll get confused. Each day's circuit selects three exercises from each of the three categories (upper body, lower body, abs), so the exercises will vary from day to day and keep you challenged.

Before you start doing any of the exercises that follow, we recommend that you read through this entire chapter, taking note of the instructions and illustrations for each exercise. You don't want to have to repeatedly stop and read during your workout.

Your circuit will always follow this format:

Cardio	2 minutes (This is your mandatory warm-up)
Lower body	1 minute
Upper body	1 minute
Abs	1 minute
Cardio	2 minutes
Lower body	1 minute
Upper body	1 minute
Abs	1 minute
Cardio	2 minutes
Lower body	1 minute
Upper body	1 minute
Abs	1 minute
Cardio	2 minutes
REPEAT THE ABOVE	
Abs	3 minutes
Stretch (cooldown)	3 minutes

Over the course of these fourteen days, try to work your way up to completing two rounds of the circuit within thirty-eight minutes, including fifteen seconds to set up between each station. If this isn't possible, don't worry—you'll still get the benefits so long as you keep moving and watch your form. These fourteen days are just the beginning, and if you stick with the BBC program, you will be doing circuits for a long time to come. So for now, keep up a good pace, but above all be mindful of how you do the exercises.

How Hard Should I Work?

Researchers investigating the link between exercise and longevity have studied the beneficial effects of pushing your limits during circuit training instead of "sandbagging it," which means not working as hard as you can. They found that higher-intensity workouts are more successful at reducing stress than moderate ones. So giving your all during BBC Circuit Training not only builds toned muscles and keeps you challenged, but also helps you destress and rejuvenate your body.

Circuit A

JUMP ROPE: 2 MINUTES

Jump rope or simulate jumping rope. As you jump, keep your spine straight and your abs slightly contracted, your neck long and your chin slightly tucked. Lift your knees as high as possible for added cardio benefit. Be sure to land on your toes.

Alternate: If you don't have a jump rope, simulate jumping rope or do jumping jacks instead. If you have knee problems, march in place, lifting your knees as high as possible.

PLIÉ SQUATS: 1 MINUTE (targets inner thighs and glutes)

• Stand with your feet apart, slightly wider than your hips, with your toes pointing outward.
• Bend your knees and lower yourself, keeping your back straight, and your abs slightly contracted.
• Straighten your knees and return to starting position.

Advanced: Hold a 5-pound weight (or its equivalent) with both hands, and raise the weight out in front of you to chest level while squatting down.

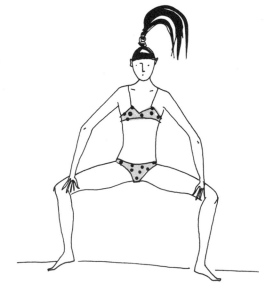

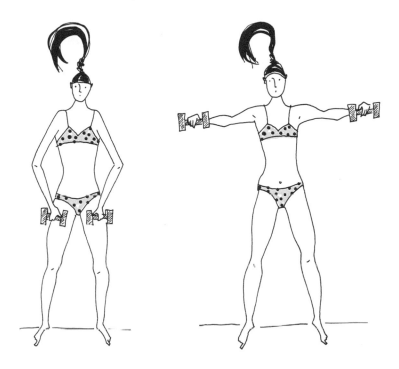

BENT ELBOW RAISES: 1 MINUTE (targets shoulders and biceps)
- Take a weight in each hand and stand with your feet
  hip-width apart, knees slightly bent. Your elbows should be bent
  at a 45-degree angle at your waist. Your palms holding the weights
  should be facing in.
- Keeping your elbows bent, raise your arms to shoulder level, and
  then lower to starting position.

SLOW BICYCLES: 1 MINUTE (targets upper and lower abdominals and
obliques)
- Lie on a mat with your knees
  bent, feet hip-width apart.
- Interlace your fingers
  behind your head and lift
  your head and shoulders as
  you contract your abs, pulling
  your navel into your spine.

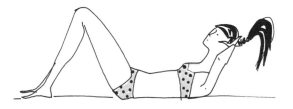

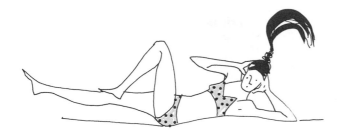

• Draw your left knee into your chest and twist your right elbow toward the left knee at the same time as you straighten your right leg, keeping it a few inches off the floor.

• Return to the center.

• Repeat on the opposite side, and keep alternating sides for 1 minute.

JUMP ROPE: 2 MINUTES

LATERAL LUNGES: 1 MINUTE
(targets outer hamstrings and glutes)

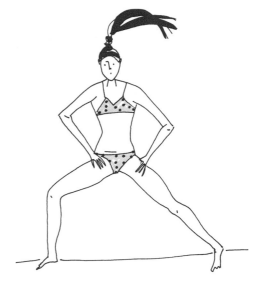

• Stand with your feet 2 to 3 feet apart, depending upon the length of your legs.

• Bend your right knee as you shift your weight to the right. Your chest leans forward as you squeeze your glutes and tilt them slightly backward so they project out behind you.

• Come all the way back up to stand in the center.

• Switch to the left and keep alternating sides for 1 minute.

Advanced: Hold a single weight with both hands, and carry the weight with you as you move from side to side.

TRICEPS DIPS: 1 MINUTE (targets triceps and core muscles)

• Sit on the edge of a chair, your hands at your sides, palms facing down and positioned directly beneath shoulders. Grip the edge of the seat with your fingertips.

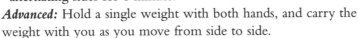

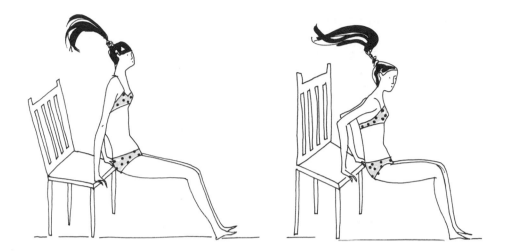

- Bend your elbows and lower yourself down and off the seat of the chair, keeping your back close to the edge.
- Straighten your arms and return to starting position. Remember, the lift comes from your arm muscles (triceps), not your legs.

BENT KNEE ROLL-UPS: 1 MINUTE (targets core muscles)
- Lie on the ground with your knees bent and your feet on the floor, hip-width apart.
- Float your arms overhead and lower them behind you. Your palms are facing up and your hands are 6 inches off the floor.
- Raise your arms straight overhead and then contract your abs, peeling your upper body off the mat, bringing your arms down in front of you. Keep your knees bent and your feet firmly planted.

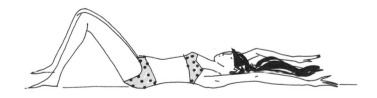

- Come fully up to a seated position, then roll back down slowly, lowering your spine gently, vertebra by vertebra—the slower the better.

Tip: Try not to use momentum to roll up. Instead, allow your core muscles to do the work. Shaking abs are okay!

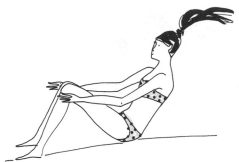

JUMP ROPE: 2 MINUTES

LEG RAISES: 1 MINUTE (targets thighs and glutes)
- Stand facing a wall, feet about 1 foot away, with your palms resting against the wall at about shoulder height. There should be a slight bend in your elbows.
- Lift your left leg slightly to the side and rotate your toes to the left.
- Keeping your toes facing left, lift your leg up and back, approximately 1 foot away from your body. Then lower to starting position. Repeat for 30 seconds.
- Switch to your right leg for the remaining 30 seconds.

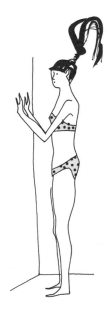
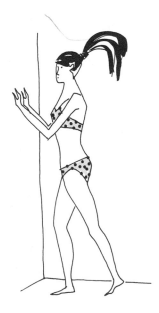

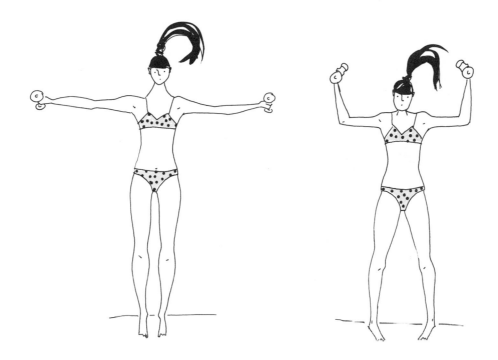

SHOULDER-LEVEL BICEPS CURLS: 1 MINUTE (targets biceps, shoulders)
- Pick up your weights and stand with your feet hip-width apart, knees slightly bent.
- Extend your arms out to the sides at shoulder height, palms facing up.
- Bend your elbows and curl the weights in toward your shoulders.
- Return to starting position and repeat.

Bikini Tip ⋯⋯⋯⋯⋯⋯⋯⋯⋯⋯⋯⋯⋯⋯⋯⋯⋯⋯⋯⋯⋯⋯⋯⋯⋯⋯

If you need to take a break, take it, but sit still for no more than 3 minutes between sets. Waiting longer allows your muscles to cool down and your heart rate to drop, weakening the benefits of the exercises.

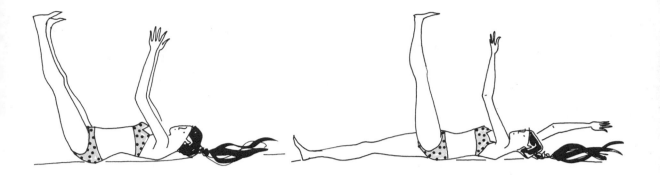

DEAD BUG: 1 MINUTE (targets core, arms, and legs)
- Lie on your back with your legs extended straight overhead, your feet flexed and in line with your hips.
- Extend your arms straight overhead, your palms facing in toward each other and in line with your shoulders.
- Lower your right arm and your right leg, until they hover 1 inch above the floor.
- Raise your arm and leg back to starting position, and repeat the motion for 30 seconds.
- Switch sides and repeat for the remaining 30 seconds.

JUMP ROPE: 2 MINUTES

REPEAT ALL OF THE ABOVE STARTING WITH PLIÉ SQUATS

3-MINUTE ABS: TRADITIONAL CRUNCHES WITH ALTERNATE LEG EXTENSIONS (targets upper and lower abdominals)

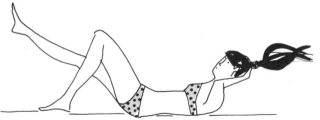

- Lie on your back with your knees bent, your feet on the floor, hip-width apart. Interlace your hands behind your head.
- Lift your head, neck, and shoulders up off the mat, squeezing your abs and pulling your navel to your spine. As you lift your upper body, extend your

right leg; as you lower back down, bend your knee and return to the original position. Repeat on the other side.
• Continue crunches for three minutes, alternating extensions on the right and left legs.

3-MINUTE STRETCH

• Sit on the mat with your legs extended out in front of you and to-gether, your feet flexed and your spine straight, with your shoulders relaxed down.
• Inhale your arms straight up and overhead.
• Now exhale, folding forward, with the crown of your head reaching toward your toes, so that you are looking down at your thighs, knees, or calves. You can always hold a towel or belt looped around your feet to help reach your toes and really stretch all the muscles running along the back side of your body, from your heels to your neck.
• Hold for 1 minute, and then slowly roll up to the starting position.

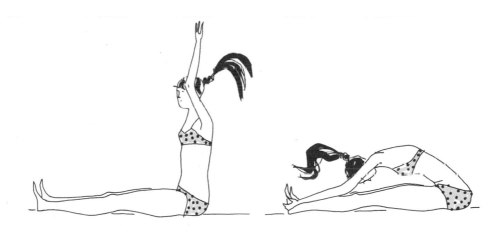

- With your legs straight and together, your feet flexed, and your spine tall, bend your right knee and draw the sole of your right foot up to the inner thigh of your extended left leg. Inhale your arms up and overhead.
- Exhale, folding forward over your extended left leg. Hold for 30 seconds.
- Repeat with the right leg extended, bringing the sole of your left foot to rest against the inner thigh of your right leg and folding forward over your extended right leg. Hold for 30 seonds.
- Now sit in a cross-legged position and straighten your arms overhead, palms facing up with your fingertips interlaced. Bend to the left and hold for the count of 15 seconds. Repeat on the opposite side.

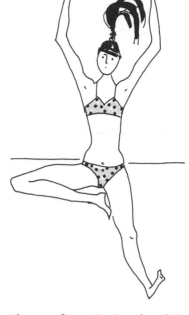

Remember: ··

Do not count reps. Repeat each exercise for the allotted time, aiming for perfect form. Also remember, whenever you are doing any kind of exercise, to never lock your knees or elbows. Keep them slightly soft but controlled, to prevent joint injury.

··

Circuit B

JUMP ROPE: 2 MINUTES (If you have knee trouble, march in place, lifting your knees as high as possible.)

REVERSE LUNGES: 1 MINUTE (targets glutes and hamstrings)
- Stand with your back toward the wall, about 18 inches away.
- Your feet should be planted flat on the ground. Step your left foot back so the heel touches the wall.
- Bend both your knees, leaning slightly forward as your hips shift back toward the wall, as if you were in the process of sitting down. Do not actually touch the wall with your back or hips.
- Come up to standing position. Repeat for 30 seconds.
- Switch sides.

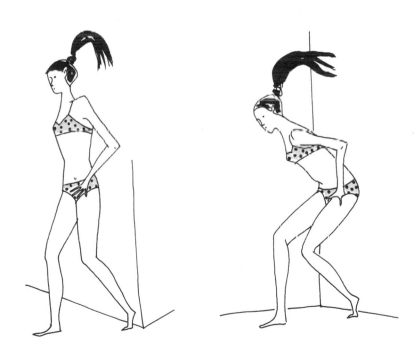

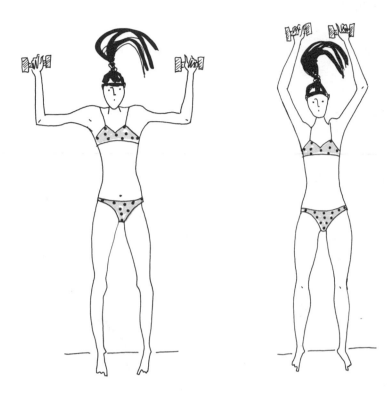

OVERHEAD PRESS: 1 MINUTE (targets upper back, front, and middle shoulders)

- Stand with your feet hip-width apart, knees slightly bent. Hold a weight in each hand.
- Bend your elbows and raise them up and out to the sides, so they form right angles with your body. Your elbows should be in line with your shoulders, with your palms facing forward.
- Keeping your palms facing out, raise your arms overhead so that the weights lightly touch. Make sure you keep your elbows slightly bent.
- Now lower your weights so that your elbows again form 90-degree angles.
- Repeat.

SIDE EXTENSIONS: 1 MINUTE (targets core, shoulders, and abdominal obliques)
- Stand with your feet hip-width apart, knees slightly bent.
- Hold a single weight (3 to 5 pounds) with both hands.
- Extend your arms and the weight overhead, keeping your elbows slightly bent.
- Now lean to the right, tilting your body and the weight slightly forward, as far as you can.
- Return to center starting position and repeat on the left.

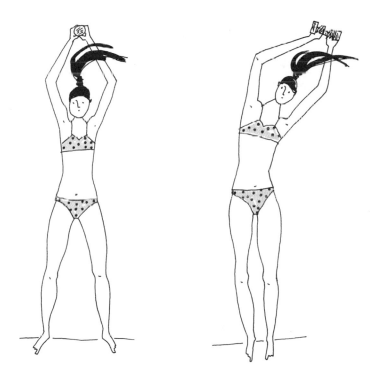

JUMP ROPE: 2 MINUTES

WALL SITS: 1 MINUTE (targets hamstrings and glutes)

- Stand with your legs hip-width apart and lean back against a wall.
- Sit down as if you were in an imaginary chair. Make sure your knees are in line with your hips, your knees directly over your ankles and hip-width apart. Hold for 1 minute. *Advanced:* Squeeze a rolled towel or book between your knees to target the inner thighs as well.

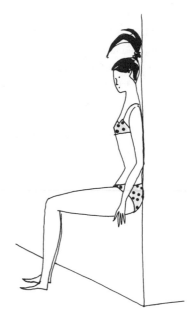

STANDING TRICEPS KICKBACKS: 1 MINUTE (target any part of the triceps simply by rotating your wrist to different angles.)

- Stand with your feet flat on the floor, shoulder-width apart, knees slightly bent to take the pressure off your back. Place your right hand on the back of a chair or counter for balance and hold a weight in your left hand.

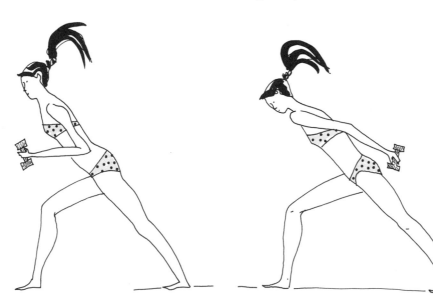

- Bend at your hip joints and lean forward so your upper body is at a 30- to 45-degree angle and step back with your left leg. Pull your left arm back so it's parallel to your body, and bend your elbow so that your lower arm forms a right angle.
- Straighten your left arm, pushing the weight back to contract your triceps. Your elbow stays attached to your side as much as possible throughout the motion.
- Now bend your elbow to return your arm to the starting position. Repeat for 30 seconds, and then switch to the other side.

To work the inner triceps: Hold the weight with your palm facing straight to the floor.

To work the middle and outer part of the muscle: Turn the weight so your palm is facing your body.

TRADITIONAL CRUNCHES: 1 MINUTE (targets abdominals)
- Lie on the mat with your knees bent and touching one another and your feet firmly planted.
- Interlace your fingers behind your head and lift your head and shoulders as you contract your abs, pulling your navel into your spine.
- Release the adbominal contraction as your lower your head and shoulders back to the mat.
- Repeat.

Advanced: Perform the same movement, but this time, lift your feet off the mat and straighten and extend your legs as you do the crunch. Then release the abdominal contraction and lower your feet, head, and shoulders to the starting position.

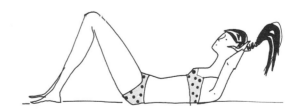

JUMP ROPE: 2 MINUTES

HIP ROTATORS: 1 MINUTE (targets glutes and hip flexors)

- Lie on your right side with your knees bent at a 90-degree angle, as if you were sitting in a chair. Your knees are in line with your hips, and your ankles in line with your knees. Prop your head up on your right hand, and make sure that your left leg is stacked directly on top of the right. Flex both feet.

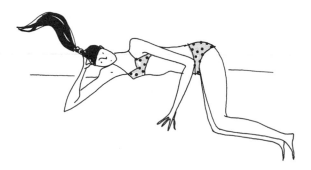

- Making sure that your knees continue to touch, lift the lower part of your left leg. The top of your left knee will be touching the right knee and your foot will be up in the air.
- Now rotate your left hip socket outward so that your knee lifts up into the air and your left foot comes down to touch the right foot (toe to toe). Then lower your knee back down to the previous position.
- Repeat for 30 seconds and then switch sides.

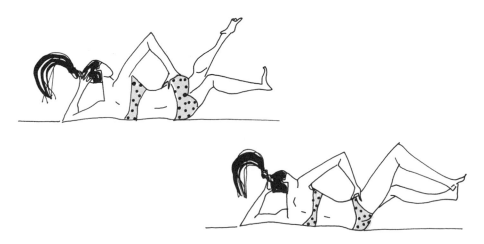

PUSH-UPS: 1 MINUTE (targets chest, shoulders, and biceps)

- Get down on the mat on your hands and knees. Your palms are flat on the mat, slightly wider than your shoulders, your arms straight. Extend your legs straight behind you, hip-width apart, with the balls of your feet pressed down on the mat.
- Bend your arms and lower your chest toward the floor, keeping your core engaged and your back straight by pulling your navel toward your spine throughout.
- Push back up into the starting position and repeat.

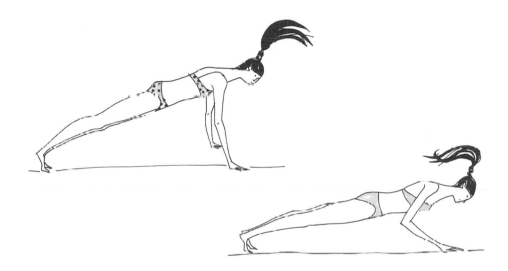

Beginner's alternative: Position your arms in the same way, but rest on your knees, your feet lifted behind you, so that your body forms a diagonal line from your knees to your head. Tighten your abs as you exhale and lower yourself down to the point where the tip of your nose touches the floor, but no further. Inhale and push back up, straightening your arms.

Elevated alternative (works the same muscles, especially the chest): Lie facedown with a chair near your feet. Raise your legs and place the top of your toes on the front edge of the seat. With your hands planted on the floor, shoulder-width apart, raise and lower yourself as you would for a regular push-up.

UPPER BODY TWISTS: 1 MINUTE (targets obliques, sides of abs)
- Sit on a mat or rug with your knees bent and your feet planted on the floor, hip-width apart.
- Lean back slightly so your back is at a 45-degree angle.
- With your left hand, reach across your body to the right side of your knees, twisting your torso to the right as if you were grabbing something. Then reach across your body with your right hand, twisting your torso to the left. Be sure to maintain your back's 45-degree angle. Keep repeating, alternating sides.

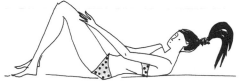

JUMP ROPE: 2 MINUTES

REPEAT ALL OF THE ABOVE STARTING WITH REVERSE LUNGES.

3-MINUTE ABS (targets lower abs)
- Lie on your back and, keeping your legs straight, raise them so they're over your hips.
- Now cross your feet at the ankles and interlace your hands behind your head.

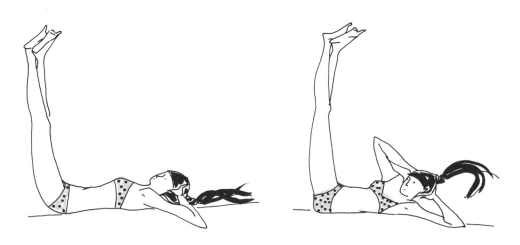

- Use your abdominal muscles to lift up and reach your right elbow over to the opposite knee, keeping your legs straight and perpendicular to your body the entire time.
- Come back to center and then reach your left elbow to the right knee. Keep repeating, alternating sides.

3-MINUTE STRETCH

- Lie on your back with your right knee bent and your right foot planted on the floor. Your left leg is raised straight up over your hips, foot flexed.
- Loop a towel or belt around the sole of your flexed foot and draw your straight leg in toward your chest, keeping your shoulders and head on the ground. Make sure your foot is flexed, with the heel pushing out and away from you. Hold for 1 minute.

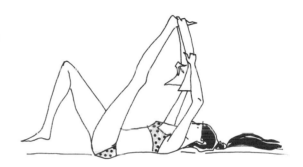

- Lower your left leg and repeat on your right side. Hold for 1 minute.
- Now stand with your feet together and knees slightly bent. Inhale your arms up and overhead, and take hold of your left wrist with your right hand. Exhale as you lean your body over to the right. Hold for 30 seconds. Repeat on the opposite side, holding the right wrist with the left hand and leaning to the left. Hold for 30 seconds.

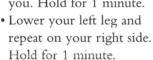

Remember to check your level of weight to make sure you're getting the optimum workout. Most people underestimate their strength; so if you can easily do 10 reps with the weight you're using, kick it up a notch until you reach a weight where you feel challenged.

Circuit C

JUMP ROPE: 2 MINUTES (Remember, you can do jumping jacks or simulated jumping rope if you like. If your knees bother you, simply march in place, lifting your knees as high as possible.)

STATIONARY LUNGES: 1 MINUTE (targets hamstrings, calves)
- Stand with your feet together and step your right foot forward, about 3 feet. Bend your right knee, lowering yourself until your left knee almost touches the floor. Your right knee should remain directly above your right ankle.

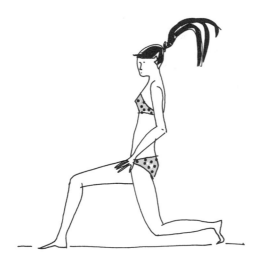

- Now straighten both your legs and step back to starting position. Repeat for 30 seconds, and then switch sides.

Advanced: Add a 3- to 5-pound weight in each hand.

BICEPS CURLS: 1 MINUTE (targets biceps)

- Stand with your feet planted firmly on the floor, holding a 3- to 5-pound weight in each hand. Your legs are hip-width apart, your abs contracted, and your spine in a neutral position.
- Keeping your upper arms parallel to your body, inhale as you bring the weights up to your shoulders slowly and evenly, with palms facing up, for a full contraction. Throughout the movement, keep your arms shoulder-width apart and make sure that your arms remain stationary in order to focus the workout on the biceps.
- Exhale as you slowly bring your lower arms back down for a full stretch.

Advanced: For added intensity, shift your elbows 1 inch away from your waist and proceed with the exercise.

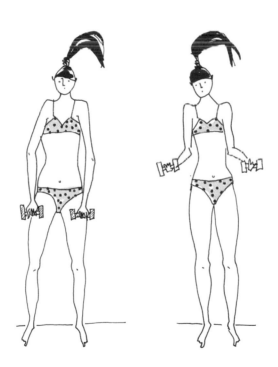

CRISS-CROSS ABS: 1 MINUTE (targets obliques)

- Lie down on the mat, with your legs straight and your arms extended overhead.
- Bend your right knee and place your right foot on the mat, next to your left knee. Place your left hand next to your left hip, palm facing down.
- Rotate your left leg outward so your toes point to the left.
- Keeping your knee straight, contract your abs as you lift your left leg and right hand so they meet over your midsection.
- Lower and repeat for 30 seconds, and then switch sides.

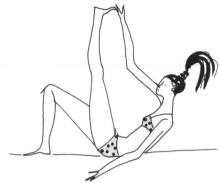

JUMP ROPE: 2 MINUTES

INNER THIGH LIFTS: 1 MINUTE (targets inner and outer thighs)

- Lie on your left side with your knees bent, as if you were sitting in a chair. Your knees should be in line with your hips, and your ankles

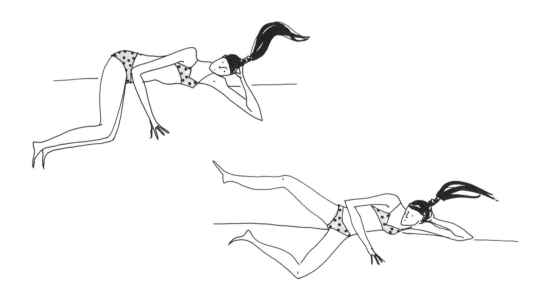

in line with your knees. Prop up your head in your left hand, and make sure that the right leg is stacked directly on top of the left. Flex both feet.

- Lift your bent right leg up about 18 inches and then lower. Lift and lower this leg for 30 seconds, and then repeat on your opposite leg.

UPRIGHT ROWS: 1 MINUTE (targets shoulder, biceps, and trapezius)
- Stand with your feet hip-width apart and your knees slightly bent. Hold a 3- to 5-pound weight in each hand, palms facing back.
- Bend your elbows and bring the weights straight up to shoulder height. Your elbows extend straight out to the sides; your palms remain facing down to work the biceps and the forearm muscles.
- Lower and repeat.

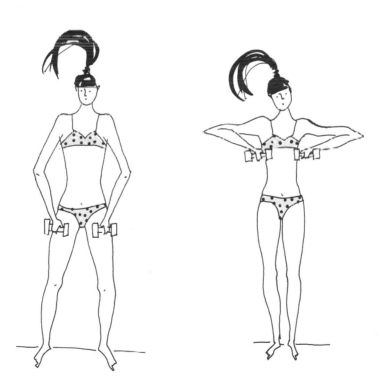

SIDE CRUNCHES: 1 MINUTE (targets obliques)

- Lie on your back with your knees bent, and your knees and toes touching.
- Drop both knees to the floor on the right. Your back and shoulders should remain flat on the floor, giving you a nice twist along your spine.
- Interlace your fingers behind your head, and then lift your head, neck, and shoulders straight up off the mat. Don't pull on your neck and head with your hands; instead, use your abdominal muscles to do the movement. Lift and lower for 30 seconds.
- Return to starting position with your knees in the center, and then drop them over to the left. Repeat on your left side for 30 seconds.

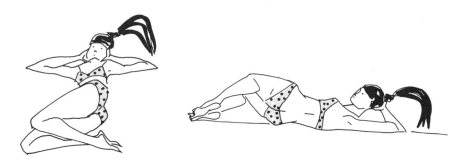

JUMP ROPE: 2 MINUTES

SHUFFLING SQUATS: 1 MINUTE (targets inner and outer thighs, glutes, calves, plus cardio benefits)

- Stand with your feet together and your toes touching. Take a large step to the right with your right foot, keeping the left foot stationary and bending both knees into a squat.
- Now bring your right foot back to center to meet your left foot. Then step to the left with your left foot, keeping the right foot stationary and bending both knees into a squat. Bring your left foot back to center to meet your right foot. Keep alternating both sides.

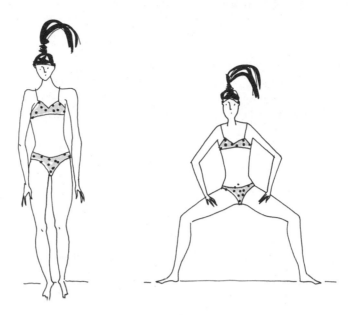

Advanced: Add a hop between the side squats by propelling yourself upward when you bring your feet back to center. This intensifies the cardio benefit.

CRISS-CROSS ARMS: 1 MINUTE (targets shoulders and lats)

- Stand with your feet hip-width apart, your knees slightly bent.
- Holding a weight in each hand, raise your arms straight out in front of your chest, elbows slightly bent.
- Now criss-cross your arms, keeping your fists close to one an-other and your wrists level rather than bent up or down. Lower only when it's time to move on to the next exercise.

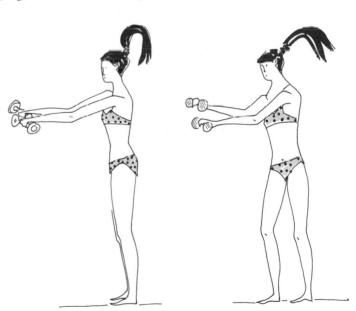

PLANK: 1 MINUTE (targets full body: core, shoulders, arms, and legs)

- Lie facedown on the mat with your hands directly beneath your shoulders, your fingers widespread, and your palms pressing into the floor. Your legs are extended hip-width apart with your toes curled under. Your body forms a straight line from head to heels.
- Now push your body up and away from the floor. If you need assistance, support yourself on your knees to come into a full plank position. Bring your arms to full extension, with your hands still in line with your shoulders. Be sure to gaze downward, so your neck is straight. Your legs are extended straight and long behind you, toes curled under, heels reaching away from you.
- Pull your navel to your spine to engage your abdominals, and hold for 1 minute.

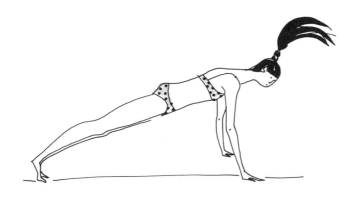

Advanced: As you're holding the plank position, lift your right leg 12 inches off the floor and hold for 30 seconds. Lower and repeat with your left leg.

JUMP ROPE: 2 MINUTES

REPEAT ALL OF THE ABOVE STARTING WITH STATIONARY LUNGES.

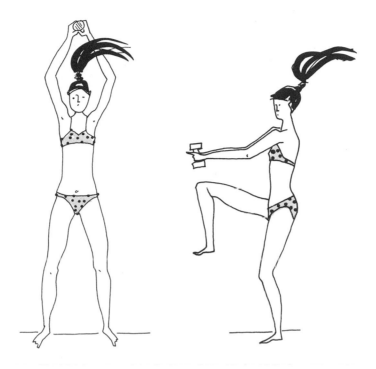

3-MINUTE ABS: KNEE LIFTS (targets abs and shoulders)
- Stand with your feet hip-width apart, holding a single weight with both hands.
- Extend your arms up overhead, keeping a slight bend in your elbows.
- Now lift your right knee as you lower your arms so the weight and your knee meet just above hip height.
- Lower your right knee, and raise your arms back up overhead.
- Repeat on your left side and keep alternating legs until the 3 minutes are up.

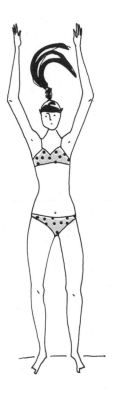

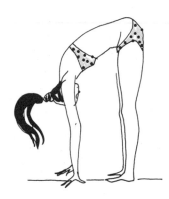

3-MINUTE STRETCH

- Stand with your feet planted shoulder-width apart. Inhale your arms up and overhead.
- Exhale as you fold forward, the crown of your head reaching toward the earth, and plant your palms on the floor, if that's possible, in line with your shoulders.
- Shift your weight slightly forward so that the weight of your body is felt equally in your toes and heels. Hold for 1 minute.
- Straighten back up and then spread your legs *wider* than shoulder-width. Fold over again, so the crown of your head is pointing toward the floor.
- Bend your right knee into a light lunge and walk your hands over to the right side of your body, stretching the left side. Hold for 1 minute. Straighten your leg and return to center, then bend your left knee, walking your hands over to the left, stretching your right side. Hold for 1 minute.

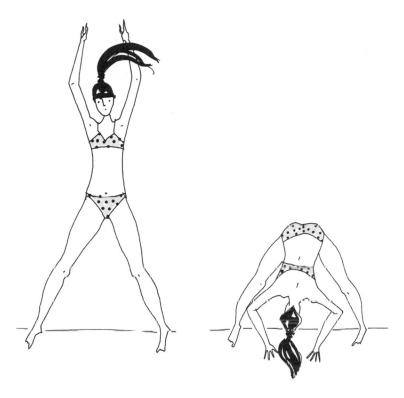

Keys to Performing Circuits

Now that you understand how the circuit works, here are some points to keep in mind during your workout to minimize stress on your body and maximize your results.

- Keeping perfect form with moderate weights will create more gains than overloading the muscles with heavy weights. So don't be afraid to start light—beginners should start with about 3 pounds—and work your way up, maxing at 8 pounds.
- Breathe properly with continuous and evenly timed inhalations and exhalations. You want to inhale through your nose to allow your nostrils to filter the air, and exhale through your mouth to expel air fully from your body. Never hold your breath!
- Perform each exercise slowly and smoothly with full range of motion and full control. The good extension on each rep—that is, the return to the starting position—is just as important as the good

contraction, so be sure both movements are done deliberately and with focus.

- Always make sure you are hydrated before starting any exercise to help your body recover quickly and prevent the harmful effects of dehydration. Drink two 8-ounce glasses of water two hours before you exercise, a glass right before you start, and a glass during your workout whenever you feel the need.
- Work to the point where you feel challenged, but do not advance too quickly in terms of increasing weights; in doing so you risk injury. A good rule of thumb is to increase your weights by no more than 10 percent per week. Heavy weights are not needed for these exercises.
- Pay attention to which muscles are being trained. If you follow the BBC circuits exactly, you'll avoid duplicating a movement in a single workout. Overtraining any muscle can slow you down and lead to injury.
- Be sure to warm up and cool down. Warming up increases blood flow to your muscle tissue and gives you a more efficient workout. The daily yoga and walks that are part of BBC are great warm-ups for circuit training. Cooling down after exercising restores your heart to its normal rate and allows your body to flush out the wastes produced by exercise that can add to muscle soreness and fatigue. You can cool down by doing the recommended stretching, or by walking a little.

Bikini Tip

Believe it or not, there is a right and a wrong way to stretch. Here's how to get the most out of your cooldowns:

- First imagine the muscles you are going to stretch. Inhale and then exhale to relax them. The longer your exhale, the more your muscles will relax.
- Hold each stretch for 30 seconds to a minute as directed, breathing deeply and taking long exhales.

- If you experience muscle or joint pain, try the sports injury prescription: RICE—Rest, Ice, Compress, and Elevate. Call your doctor if this treatment, plus stopping moderate to strenuous exercising, does not relieve symptoms within two or three days.

• Never exercise on an empty stomach. Be sure to eat one to three hours before working out, and make sure you eat again within two hours after exercising.

Our Favaorite Circuit Training Playlist

At Bikini Bootcamp, our favorite music selections fire up our campers' spirits and keep them going during a brisk circuit training workout. We suggest you rev up your energy and keep it high throughout your session by sweating to your own musical favorites—tunes that make you feel like kicking some serious butt! For real BBC atmosphere, try any of the following songs that are in heavy rotation on our playlist:

1. Shaggy, "Mr. Lover"
2. Will Smith, "Miami"
3. Gabin, "Into My Soul"
4. Gorillaz, "Feel Good, Inc."
5. Pras Michel, "Ghetto Supastar"
6. Gwen Stefani, "Hollaback Girl"
7. Paperboy, "Ditty"
8. Missy Elliott, "4 My People"
9. Pussycat Dolls, "Don't Cha"
10. Outkast, "Way You Move"
11. Trick Daddy, "Take It to da House"
12. Sérgio Mendes, "Oh Ariaio"
13. Mary J. Blige, "Family Affair"
14. Sean Paul, "Get Busy"
15. Usher, "Yeah"

On the Road and in the Office

You don't have to blow off your BBC circuit just because you're on the road or having a crazy week at work. Use what's at hand to tone your muscles, burn calories, and jump-start your energy level. A chair, desk, and a drawer to hold some water bottles and sneakers are all you need to convert your office or cubicle into your portable gym. For more tips, see the office circuit routine we've laid out for you in Part IV.

CHAPTER 2

Core Strengthening

The body is a sacred garment.
—*Martha Graham*

When most of us try on our bathing suits at the beginning of the summer, we immediately start fretting about that most notorious of female trouble spots: the tummy. After a long winter of sitting around indoors, it's not surprising that your belly might be less than taut. The BBC core strengthening routines, performed every other day, are designed to zap that belly-fat and give you a trim, toned midsection along with a killer set of abs that will form the centerpiece of your new bikini body. And, they do so in an astonishingly brief amount of time.

Most people assume that toning your abs is a grueling process, but it doesn't have to be. Creating a lean, taut torso is not a matter of exercise *quantity* but *quality*—the right exercise done with the right form. In the past the answer was crunches, but crunches work only the *top* layer of the abdominal muscles—and as you'll see, your abs are just one of many muscle groups that are responsible for your shape around the middle. True to its name, core strengthening targets all the muscles of the core—from your back to your sides to your hips to your glutes. As a result, our core workouts deliver not only amazing definition in your abs, but slimmer hips, buttocks, and upper thighs. As you strengthen your back, you'll improve your posture and actually appear taller and slimmer—even if you don't lose a single pound! Best of all, you'll see any belly-fat melt away so when you slip on that bikini, you'll have a trim, tight waistline that emphasizes the right curves rather than the wrong ones.

The benefits of core strengthening, however, go far beyond getting a better shape. Toning your torso not only improves your posture, it also protects you against backache and injury. Your core is the center of your body, and if its muscles are weak, it's difficult for the rest of your body to work effectively, because other muscles have to pick up the slack. The result is not only a thicker middle, a sagging butt, and a hunched posture, but also an aching back, thighs, legs, and feet. And who wants that? So we encourage you to think beyond achieving that flat tummy you can bounce a dime off of (though our workouts deliver exactly that) and recognize that in strengthening all the muscles of your torso, you are supporting *everything* you do with your body. Then, you will be truly fit to the core.

The muscles of the core include:

The transverse abdominis: The deepest layer of abdominal muscle, the transverse abdominis is your natural girdle, because it wraps around the abdomen to support your internal organs as well as your spine. When you activate the transverse abdominis through core exercises, you stimulate neural activity in the multifidus, a deep extensor muscle along the spine that attaches to the vertebrae and sacrum (the five fused bones at the end of the spine) and helps keep your posture erect.

The sartorius: The longest muscle in your body, the sartorius cuts diagonally across the quadriceps (the muscle group on the front of the thigh). The sartorius assists with most hip movement, especially hip rotation, so if it's weak, the quadriceps are forced to rotate inward to support your knee. This pulls on your hips and throws off pelvic alignment. Once you activate this muscle, your quadriceps can re-align, which protects your knees and also strengthens and sculpts your thighs.

The erector spinae: Three layers of muscle form the erector spinae, which run along both sides of the entire length of your spine, from the base of the skull to the sacrum, and help you maintain an erect posture as well as keep the spine both mobile and stable. If these muscles are weak, you feel tired when standing and have difficulty staying upright and aligned, which can lead to back pain—not to mention an unflattering slouch!

The psoas: This muscle connects your lower lumbar back to the back of your thighbone and is responsible for moving your hips. If it's overly tight, the psoas pulls on the vertebrae and connective tissue, creating tension along all the muscles that connect to the pelvis. It also causes the top of your pelvis to pull forward, putting pressure on the lower back so you can't maintain proper spinal alignment.

The piriformis: Running horizontally under your glutes, the piriformis attaches at the top of your thighbone to rotate your hips outward. If the piriformis is stronger than other muscles in this area—such as your inner thighs and psoas—your hips become imbalanced, either swaying when you walk or dropping one hip lower than the other. Imbalance in your hips can create pelvic instability, which can cause lower back pain.

The gluteal muscles: Three muscles make up the gluteal muscles, also known as the buttocks, butt, or rear end: the gluteus maximus, gluteus minimus, and gluteus medius. In addition to a less than shapely posterior, weak gluteal muscles can lead to lower back pain, and difficulty climbing stairs or even getting up from a chair. Our core strength workouts will ensure that your derriere is firm and bikini-ready with a little lift in all the right places.

The external and internal oblique muscles: Located on either side of your abdomen, the external obliques allow you to twist and turn your torso. The internal obliques are located just inside the left and right hipbones and work in tandem with the externals to give you movement. Weak obliques cause lower back pain and a flabby midsection. If you have love handles—even little ones—or recoil in horror at the roll that creeps over the edge of your bathing suit near your hips, these are the muscles to work.

The trapezius: The large muscle that makes up your upper and middle back stabilizes the thoracic (middle) spine. When you contract this muscle, you keep your shoulders pulled down and back, which helps maintain proper head and neck alignment and opens your chest for expanded breathing capacity. A toned trapezius not only gives you a shapely back, it also prevents rounded shoulders and droopy posture. Is there anything less sexy than walking around all hunched over? We don't think so. It's bad for your appearance *and* your body.

Your core muscles include not only the abdominal and back muscles described above, but also other muscles found deep in the pelvic floor and hips. Many of these muscles can't be seen or even felt as they do their work during the course of your everyday activity. Yet they all must work together to stabilize your spine and midsection while you are active, and any core workout you do must contain a balanced approach. For example, your abdominal muscles function in opposition to—and together with— your back muscles. So, if you work your abs without working your back and glutes, you are setting yourself up for core imbalance that can lead to future aches and pains. Or if you work your abs and glutes without paying attention to the classic imbalance that causes chronic slouching—weak upper and middle back muscles that are often combined with overly tight chest muscles—you won't get the results, or the posture, you want. The BBC core strengthening routines help you maintain equal tension in all the opposing muscle groups that form your core to create strength, stability, and symmetry throughout your torso.

We've provided you with two different core strengthening series—Series A and Series B—which give you enough variety to prevent boredom, but not so much as to overcomplicate your workout. Each of the two series takes about twenty minutes and consists of several exercises done in succession, with few repetitions, because you will be paying close attention to alignment and form. Our two core series are inspired by the Pilates exercise system, which was developed in Germany by Joseph H. Pilates over one hundred years ago to help rehabilitate dancers after debilitating injuries. Some of the exercises in your core strengthening series will be familiar from your circuit training. That's okay—it never hurts to double up on these exercises after you've given your muscles a chance to rest!

What You'll Need

- A mat
- Comfortable clothing

We recommend that, like our Bikini Bootcampers, you don't wear shoes or sneakers during these exercises. Going barefoot allows you to point and flex your toes with greater ease.

Posture Is Important

Maintaining correct abs-and-back-strengthening posture as you perform your core series is crucial. To check your posture, stand sideways in front of a full-length mirror. Contract your abs and tuck in your tailbone slightly, but not so much that you lose the curve in your lower back. You will immediately see your abs flatten and your back lengthen and straighten. You might even appear to have grown taller! This is the posture you want to maintain while working your core. Keep those abs pulled in whether sitting or standing to ensure you're getting the maximum workout and protecting yourself from injury.

Remind yourself to hold this posture throughout your day, while driving, standing in line at the bank, or sitting at your desk. You will be strengthening your back, glutes, and abs, and even burning extra calories. As this posture becomes second nature, the exercises will become easier. Don't be surprised if people start asking if you're a dancer!

Repetitions and Frequency

You will perform one of our core series every other day, following the programs we've laid out for you. One set makes for an efficient workout, but if you have time, try to do a second set. If possible, do your core series after circuit training or yoga so you are already warmed up before working your back muscles. Even after you've completed the fourteen-day intensive BBC program and/or have reached your desired weight, shape, and fitness level, keep incorporating two core strengthening sessions into your week, performed either alone or in conjunction with circuit training and yoga for long-term health and fitness. Remember to cool down by stretching all your major muscle groups.

Less is more! New research disproves the old body-building adage that three sets of an exercise are better than one. In fact, a single set, performed well, gives you as much strength training in one-third the time. All this makes it easier to stick to your routine.

Core Strengthening Series A

CRISS-CROSS ABS (targets obliques)

- Lie down on the mat with your legs straight, your arms extended overhead.
- Bend your right knee and place your right foot on the mat.
- Place your left hand next to your left hip, palm facing down.
- Rotate your left leg outward so your toes point to the left.
- Keeping your knee straight, contract your abs as you lift your left leg and right hand toward one another, so they meet over your midsection. Lower and repeat 15 times, and then switch sides.

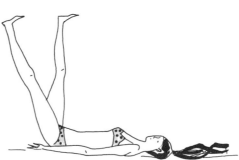

CONTROLLED LEG DROPS (targets lower abdominals)

- Lie on the mat with your arms at your sides, palms facing down, and your legs straight, hip-width apart.
- Contract your abs as you lift your legs straight up over your hips, keeping your feet flexed. Make sure your feet are directly over your hips, not over your face.
- Contract your abs, pulling your navel toward your spine.
- Lower your left leg 6 inches. Hold for the count of 3, and then bring it back to its original position overhead. Repeat 10 times on the left leg, and 10 times on the right.

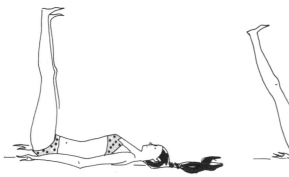

- Now lower your straight left leg 1 foot. Hold for the count of 3 and then bring it back up. Repeat 10 times on the left leg and 10 times on the right.
- Now lower your straight left leg until it hovers 1 foot *above the floor*. Hold for the count of 3. Repeat 10 times on the left leg and 10 times on the right.

DEAD BUG (targets core, arms, and legs)
- Lie on your back with your legs extended straight overhead. Keep your feet flexed and in line with your hips.
- Extend your arms straight and overhead, with your palms facing in toward one another and in line with your shoulders.
- Contract your abs as you lower your left arm and your left leg in opposite directions, until they hover 1 inch above the floor.
- Raise your arm and leg back to starting position.
- Repeat 10 times on each side.

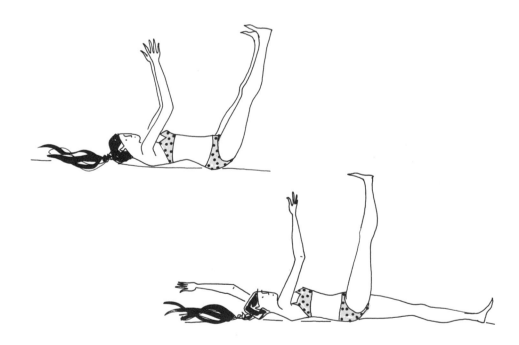

TRADITIONAL CRUNCHES (targets abdominals)
- Lie on the mat with your knees bent, feet on the floor, knees touching one another.
- Interlace your fingers behind your head and lift your head and shoulders as you contract your abs, pulling your navel into your spine.
- Release the abdominal contraction as you lower your head and shoulders back to the mat. Repeat 20 times.

Advanced: Perform the same movement, but this time lift your feet off the mat and straighten and extend your legs as you do the crunch. Then release the abdominal contraction and lower your feet, head, and shoulders to the starting position.

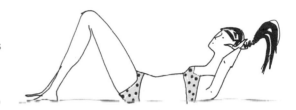

SINGLE LEG STRETCH (targets abs and thighs)
- Lie on your back with your legs straight. Inhale as you lift your head, neck, and shoulder blades up, pressing your lower back into the mat as you take hold of your left thigh or calf and draw your straight left leg in as close to your body as you can. Your right leg should remain straight but rise about a foot and a half off the floor.
- Now exhale as you release and lower your left leg at the same time that you grab onto your right leg and pull your head and right leg close together. Keep your straight left leg about a foot and a half off the floor. Repeat 10 times on each side.

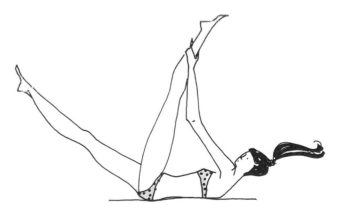

SWIMMING (Lengthens and strengthens spine, works core, and opens chest)
- Lie facedown on the mat with your legs together and extended straight. Your arms are extended straight overhead, palms on the mat.
- Contract your abs as you inhale and lift your legs and upper body, including your arms, up off the mat, making sure to keep your neck long and your gaze on the mat so you don't strain your neck.
- Now, exhale as you lift your straight left arm and straight right leg even higher, making sure to keep your legs close together. Now switch and lift your right arm and left leg.
- Repeat 10 times on each side, making quick paddling motions, as if you're swimming.

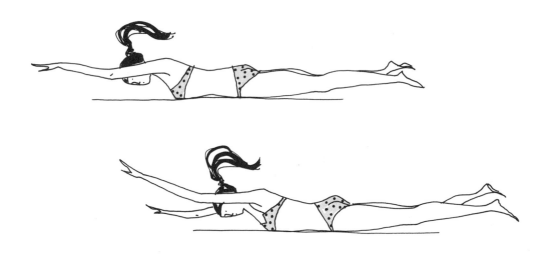

Bikini Tip ···
You can do your core series to your favorite music, as long as it has a slow tempo (85 beats per minute) that helps you execute each exercise in a slow, deliberate way, promoting control and isolation of the movement.

···

Core Strengthening Series B

SLOW BICYCLES (targets upper and lower abs and obliques)
- Lie on the mat with your knees bent, feet on the floor, hip-width apart.
- Interlace your fingers behind your head and lift your head and shoulders as you contract your abs, pulling your navel to your spine.
- Draw your left knee into your chest and twist your right elbow toward your left knee at the same time as you straighten your right leg, keeping it a few inches off the floor.
- Return to center and repeat on the other side. Alternate each side 15 times.

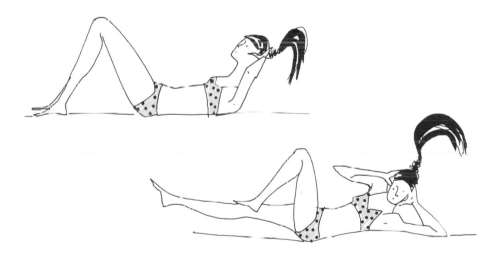

TOE DROPS (strengthens lower abs)
- Lie on your back, arms at your sides, palms facing down. Using your abdominal strength, bend your knees and draw them into your chest.

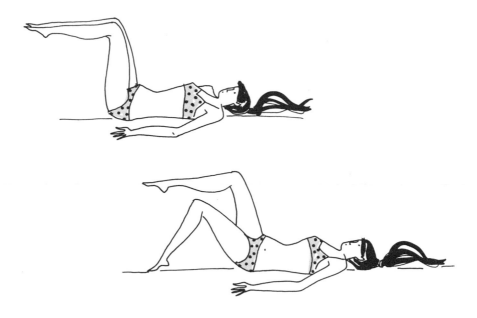

• Keeping your knees bent and your abs contracted, lower your left leg so your toes touch the ground. Repeat 25 times. Switch legs.

PLANK (targets full body, core, shoulder, arms, and legs)
• Lie facedown on the floor with your hands directly beneath your shoulders, your fingers widespread, and palms pressing into the floor. Your legs are extended hip-width apart with your toes curled under. Your body forms a straight line from head to heels.

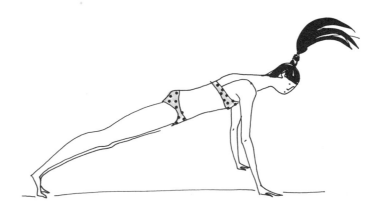

- Now push your body up and away from the floor. If you need assistance, support yourself on your knees to come into a full plank position. Bring your arms to full extension, with your hands still in line with your shoulders. Be sure to gaze downward, so your neck is straight. Your legs are extended straight and long behind you, toes curled under, heels reaching away from you.
- Keep pulling your navel to your spine to engage your abdominals and hold for 1 minute.

Advanced: As you're holding the plank position, lift your right leg 1 foot off the floor and hold for 30 seconds. Lower and repeat with your left leg.

TRADITIONAL CRUNCHES WITH ALTERNATE LEG EXTENSIONS (targets upper and lower abs)
- Lie on your back with your knees bent and feet on the floor, hip-width apart.
- Interlace your fingers behind your head, so your elbows extend out to the sides.
- Contract your abdominal muscles and lift your shoulders and neck up off the mat as you pull your navel into your spine. Make sure to keep your lower back pressed flat on the mat at all times. As you lift, extend the right leg out straight, about 6 inches above the floor.
- Lower your head and shoulders as you bend your right leg back to the starting position.
- Repeat, extending the left leg straight. Alternate legs 20 times.

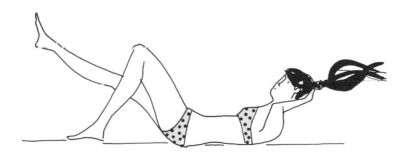

BENT KNEE ROLL-UPS (targets core)
- Lie on the floor, knees bent and feet on the floor, hip-width apart.
- Extend your arms back overhead, palms facing up.
- Lift your palms 6 inches off the floor.
- Peel your upper body off the mat, keeping your knees bent and your feet planted on the mat. Come to a seated position with a straight back.
- Roll down slowly, lowering your spine gently, vertebra by vertebra, the slower the better. Do this slowly and precisely, 10 times.

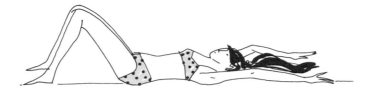

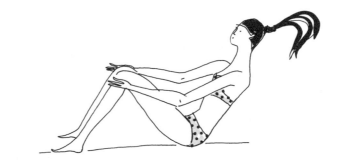

THE 100'S (strengthens and tone abs, lower back, and thighs)
- Lie down on the floor and press your lower back into the mat as you inhale and raise your legs overhead together so they are perpendicular to your torso. Your arms are straight by your sides, palms down.
- Now exhale as you lower your straight legs to the point where your lower back stays pressed down on the mat.
- Now inhale as you raise your straight arms about 6 inches off the

floor, with your fingers extended toward your toes; at the same time, engage your abs and raise your upper back, neck, and head up off the mat.

• Holding this position with your abs contracted, pump your straight arms up and down vigorously as you inhale for a count of 5 and exhale for a count of 5. Repeat this 10 times for a total count of 100.

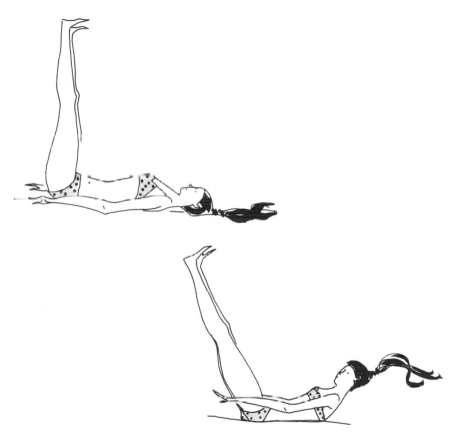

Bikini Tip

Beginners, keep your upper body, neck, and head on the mat while you do the 100's until your abs are strong enough to lift both your legs and upper body.

CHAPTER 3

Yoga

Life engenders life. Energy creates energy.
It is by spending oneself that one becomes rich.
—*Sarah Bernhardt*

Yoga is the ultimate mind/body workout and a vital part of the Bikini Bootcamp lifestyle. In Sanskrit, the word "yoga" means union of body and spirit. Five thousand years ago this venerable practice was a secret tradition, and devotees entered deep states of meditation on their way to enlightenment. Not that long ago, many people—especially those with a "gym-rat" mentality—voiced skepticism about yoga: Oh, it's just stretching and chanting "Om." Or, they viewed it as the exclusive preserve of health nuts who liked to stand on their heads and contort themselves into pretzel poses for hours. That is, until everyone came to recognize that real yoga has nothing to do with contortionist stretching and other spectacular gymnastic feats, and that its postures have the capacity, more than any bench-press, to make people look and feel younger and stronger.

The benefits of yoga are seemingly endless: it strengthens, tones, and lengthens your body for a slim and sexy look; it improves the circulation of blood and lymph to strengthen the entire cardiovascular system; it massages the internal organs; it facilitates inner calm; and it gives you a more positive sense and balanced vision of the world. We love yoga because everything it promotes, both physical and mental, is the very essence of Bikini Bootcamp. And these days, anyone can become a "yogini" with a trim and graceful shape. Your yoga workouts will help you build muscle, burn calories, and shed pounds, but they will also boost the effectiveness of your circuit training and core strengthening routines because yoga stretches and loosens muscles to the point where they can be contracted more fully during other exercises and therefore yield greater results. For example, a position like Downward-Facing Dog offers a great hamstring stretch that will enhance the benefits of your lower-body toners during circuit training and walking.

At Bikini Bootcamp, the yoga experience is ideal. We hold our classes in a large circular yoga studio with a thatched roof that allows sea breezes to waft in. Our yoginis breathe and move to the rhythm of the waves lapping onto our beach, the chirping of the birds, and, yes, the buzzing of tropical insects. Even Luna, Azul, Sol, and Pablito engage in a little Downward-Facing Dog on a daily basis. Some campers are beginners; others are more experienced and are so inspired by their surroundings that their morning practice can last up to two and a half hours! But don't panic. You don't have to perform yoga for an entire morning to get sculpted arms, perfect posture, and all the other body benefits yoga offers. We've distilled the best, most effective yoga moves into fifteen-minute Sun Salutation routines for beginner, intermediate, and advanced levels. We've stripped away some of the chanting and lengthily held postures that accompany some types of practice—so you can get more bang for your buck in a limited amount of time. Believe it or not, all you need to get that hot yoga body is fifteen minutes of Sun Salutations every morning or evening, combined with our other workouts and eating plans.

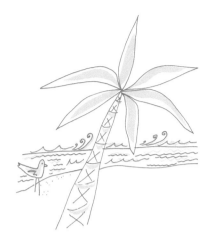

At its most basic, yoga involves moving through a progression of postures *(asanas)* while practicing breathing techniques *(pranayama)*. Yoga *asanas* are about moving, adjusting, and aligning your body, safely and according to your ability—as well as venturing beyond your comfort level so you can extend your present limits. Doing the postures *will* make you more flexible, but as we've already mentioned, the benefits go much deeper, even beyond cardiovascular endurance and toning, muscle strength, and that perky yoga butt. The breathing techniques called *pranayamas* are particularly designed to calm, balance, and energize you, so that your breath is always there for your benefit, whenever you need to cope with any challenging situation. Yoga will even prevent and help correct many muscular, skeletal, nervous system–related, or organ health problems, no matter how chronic, severe, or limiting they may be. Here are just some of yoga's terrific benefits:

- Forward bends calm the nervous system and refresh the brain.
- Twists cleanse and tone internal organs, improving digestion and

eliminating sluggishness, as well as relieve backaches, headaches, and stiff necks and shoulders.

- Restorative poses stimulate the relaxation response and conserve and restore energy, thereby improving circulation and respiration. Lying facedown is energizing, while lying face up is restful.
- Sitting poses energize the body by stimulating digestion, regulating kidney function, and promoting strength and flexibility in the back, hips, knees, neck, and shoulders.
- Balancing poses develop muscle tone, balance, strength, and agility, thereby improving coordination and concentration.
- Inverted postures and arm balances revitalize the entire body, improve circulation and gland function, and promote balance and mental clarity.

One of the many advantages of yoga is that it can be practiced in brief intervals throughout your day. The fifteen-minute sessions of yoga Sun Salutations that you will perform during BBC can fit into a crammed schedule with little disruption. Best of all, there is no goal, no competition, in yoga. Wherever you are in your practice is exactly where you should be.

The yoga you do as part of your BBC experience will also help you become a more focused and effective being who is better able to handle the challenges of her busy life. The breath-work and concentration you need for the *asanas* and *pranayamas* (breathing exercises) will help you stop fretting about the past or worrying about the future, because yoga practice calls you to be fully in the here and now. By encouraging you to move and breathe slowly, properly, and consciously, yoga helps reduce anxiety and encourages you to surrender entirely to the present. When you're in the Reverse Warrior or Crescent *asana,* for example, how can you possibly focus on anything but breathing and maintaining the posture? The greatest gift yoga brings you is the peace, balance, and clarity that results from really tuning in.

Yoga is the ideal balance between effort and surrender because it is just as important to know when to push yourself farther as when to back off from a posture. You want to work from a place that challenges you without subjecting yourself to negative stress or pain—whether this applies to the breath, the duration of your practice, the speed at which you practice the postures, or the *asanas* themselves. The idea is to stay present to the moment and discover your own balance, and, most of all, to enjoy the never-ending yoga journey.

At Bikini Bootcamp we've yet to meet a yoga skeptic or novice who wasn't hooked after only a session or two. You may not be performing your *asanas* to the sound track of the Caribbean Sea, but wherever you do your yoga, you can count on becoming hooked, too. So grab a candle, a yoga mat, and your favorite inspiring CD—it can be anything from nature sounds or waves crashing to folk music or alternative rock—and let our Sun Salutations perform their magic. There is no quicker way to feel good about your body: No matter how you felt just before beginning your daily practice, you are sure to feel ten times better afterward—refreshed, energized, grounded, and calm.

....

A word of caution: Because yoga injuries to joints and backs are on the rise, we recommend that if you do not already practice yoga, you seek out a class in your area so you are introduced properly to yoga form and practice. Yoga classes are sprouting like palm trees, in even the tiniest towns across our country. It may take sampling one or two classes at a few different studios to find the right one for you, but many studios offer free introductory sessions. Often the personality of the instructor and the energy of the class can make a huge difference. Your teacher will encourage you to also establish a home practice in addition to regular class attendance.

....

The BBC Yoga Secret: Go with the Flow

Yoga typically falls into three categories: flow yoga, alignment yoga, and gentle/restorative yoga.

Flow Yoga (Ashtanga, Vinyasa, Power Yoga): These yoga styles synchronize the breath with a progressive series of postures that are linked to produce a continuous fluid and dancelike movement. Flow yogas produce intense internal heat and a detoxifying sweat and are often labeled "Bootcamp" yogas because you get a powerful workout. Those who generally enjoy more "active" forms of exercise often prefer flow yoga because it emphasizes movement rather than simply assuming a posture and holding it for balance and alignment.

Alignment Yoga (Iyengar, Anusara): These yoga styles do not emphasize flow as much as proper alignment and are known for making use of such yoga "props" as cushions, straps, blocks, and blankets.

Hatha Yoga (Kundalini, Hatha, Yin): Generally a less strenuous yoga without linked postures, Hatha is the most commonly practiced style and emphasizes the physical aspects of yoga's spiritual path with postures and breath control.

At Bikini Bootcamp we practice Vinyasa flow yoga, which strengthens your nervous system and builds internal heat while at the same time lengthening, strengthening, and toning your body from the inside out. So be prepared to sweat! There are no peaks and valleys of energy or effort in Vinyasa yoga; only steady attention paid *in the moment* to body, mind, and breath. This is one of the reasons our yoga routine is so effective—its focused, intensive nature pushes you to get the most out of every pose.

While performing Vinyasa postures, we practice a yoga technique called *ujjayi* ("victorious") breathing. This calming and energizing breath consists of drawing air in and out of both nostrils with the glottis (the opening in your throat) partially closed so that you produce a pleasant, soft, and continuous sound as you slowly and steadily exhale and inhale through your nose. *Ujjayi* breath is often described as hearing the sound of the ocean in the back of your throat. What could be more Bikini Bootcamp than that? Learning to combine the *ujjayi* breathing pattern and the postures into a continuous fluid movement will help you build mental as well as physical stamina, which in turn will help you stick to all the other aspects of your Bikini Bootcamp program, including your new, healthy eating habits.

Each type of yoga has its benefits, so even though we focus on Vinyasa at BBC, feel free to explore the different styles in order to find one that works best for you, especially if you are new to yoga. It also can be equally important to find a teacher who inspires and motivates you to continue a consistent yoga practice beyond these two weeks that maintains your bikini body and keeps you healthy and fit at every stage of your life.

Once you're familiar and comfortable with the basic postures that comprise the easy-to-follow Sun Salutation series, you can practice them on your own. These beginner, intermediate, and advanced Sun Salutations are a great way to start your day because this particular yoga sequence revives your energy, builds heat (think cardio!), and gets your juices flowing. Plus, the repetitive motions and breathing serve as a moving meditation that delivers mind-clearing, calming benefits to center you for whatever the day brings.

The BBC Yoga Routine: Sun Salutations (Surya-namaskar)

The Sun Salutation is a total body workout, designed to stretch, expand, and contract your muscles from head to toe and give you a great kick-start in a short amount of time. It works all your major muscle groups, and when you do the sequence quickly, you increase the caloric burn. Doing the series more slowly gives you a relaxing and calming effect—a nice, restorative way to either start or end your day.

You can choose your method depending on your BBC goals, but if you're a beginner, we advise you to start out slowly to learn the postures, avoid injury, and get the hang of maintaining a steady pace and breathing pattern. As you become more accustomed to the postures and the breathwork, movement will begin to flow more naturally. One of the goals of the Bikini Bootcamp program is to always strive for maximum challenge, so no matter what your level of experience, you can aim to pick up speed and give yourself a more vigorous workout as the weeks progress.

According to Hindu mythology, the Sun Salutation series originated as a way to worship the sun, so that's why we traditionally perform this sequence early in the morning, as the sun rises. It can be done anywhere; all you need is space for your mat. We recommend that you do your Sun Salutations first thing in the morning if you can, before bathing or eating, as they will actually boost your metabolic rate so you are burning calories throughout the day.

We've provided three different sequences—one for beginning students, a second for intermediate-level yoginis, and a third for advanced practitioners. Choose the Sun Salutation sequence that addresses your level. Each series provides a graceful sequence of individual positions linked by a continuous flowing motion, and each position balances the one before, stretching the body in a complementary way. The sequences themselves do not change throughout the fourteen days of the program, but you can move up to a more challenging flow or scale back, as you desire. Remember: Yoga is not a competitive sport, and wherever you are in your practice is where you should be. As with the circuit training and core strengthening routines, the instructions that follow will not be repeated on each of the fourteen days, so you'll want to turn back to this section each day until you have memorized the sequence. You will be repeating your chosen sequence as many times as you comfortably can for fifteen minutes.

$\mathcal{S}$un $\mathcal{S}$alutation: Beginner

Start off slowly to familiarize yourself with the postures. As you become more comfortable with each pose, increase the challenge by speeding up your flow for added cardio benefits, and/or holding each pose for 5 breaths for added toning. When and if you are ready, you can move on to explore the more advanced yoga sequences.

1. Mountain Pose:
Stand with your feet together and parallel, big toes touching, and hands in front of your chest in prayer position. Your shoulder blades slide down your back, and your chin is parallel to the floor. Imagine pulling your navel into your spine. Take several deep breaths, inhaling and exhaling through your nose.

2. Hands Up: As you inhale, sweep your arms out to the sides and then up so they meet overhead. Gently arch your back and look up toward your hands, making sure your abs are slightly contracted to avoid straining your lower back.

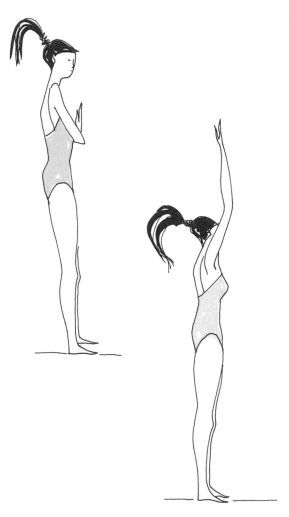

3. Forward Fold: On your next exhale, bend forward from the hinge of your hips, sweeping your arms straight out to the sides and then down so you can place your palms on the floor. Bend your knees if necessary.

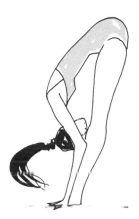

4. Flat Back: Now inhale as you lift your head and direct your gaze forward, lengthening your spine. Your fingertips can come up to your shins.

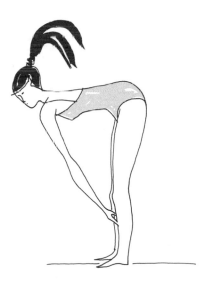

5. Plank: Exhale as you place your palms back on the floor, shoulder-width apart. Step the right leg back and then the left leg to meet the right and lower yourself into the plank (high push-up) position. Your body should form a straight line from your head to heels, with your palms directly underneath your shoulders. The crown of your head reaches away from your toes, and your abdominals are engaged by pulling your navel up to your spine. Your toes are curled under. Hold the position and inhale.

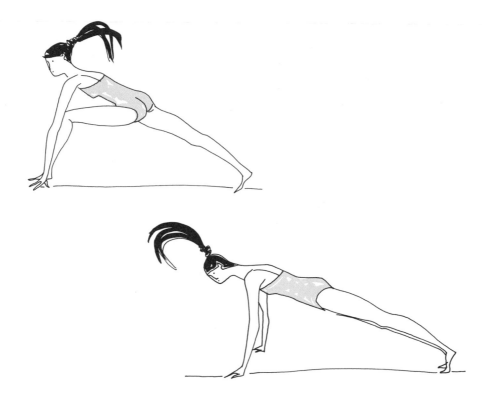

6. Stick: Now exhale as you bend your elbows and lower yourself down, as if coming down from a push-up. Your elbows stay close to your sides, hugging your ribs. Only your hands and feet should touch the floor. Modify this position if it's too difficult by lowering yourself all the way down to the mat rather than hovering just above it.

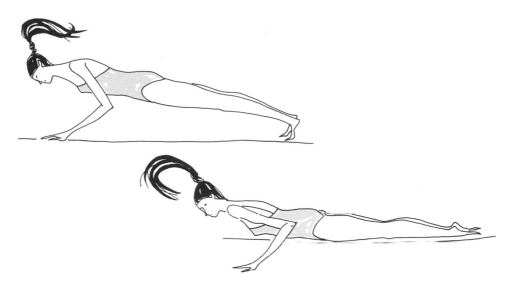

7. Upward-Facing Dog: Inhale as you straighten your arms and push your chest forward and up. Use your arms to lift your torso, but bend back only as far as feels comfortable and safe, and never drop your head all the way back. Your shoulders should be down and slightly rolled back. Now lift your legs up so that only the tops of your feet and your hands touch the floor. It's okay to keep your arms bent at the elbows.

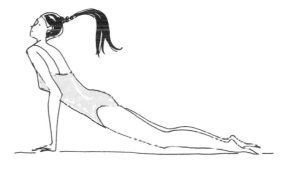

8. Downward-Facing Dog: Now exhale as you press down with your palms and lift from the hips, rolling onto the balls of your feet and pushing back and up until your legs are straight. In Downward-Facing Dog, your feet are hip-width apart, with your heels stretching down as close to the floor as possible and your hips reaching toward the sky. Lengthen your spine, and keep your hands shoulder-width apart and your neck straight.

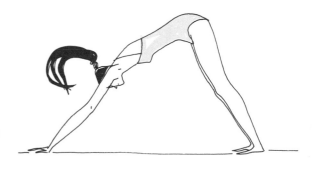

9. Lunge: Now inhale as you step the right foot forward, placing it between your hands. Take a few steps if necessary.

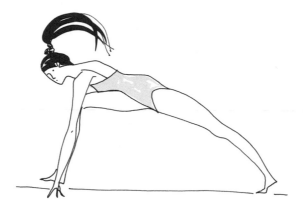

10. Forward Fold: Exhale as you bring your left foot forward so your feet are touching. Keep your palms on the floor and straighten your legs so that you are back in the Forward Fold position, your head at your knees.

11. Flat Back: Inhale as you lift your head and direct your gaze forward to stretch and lengthen your spine. Your fingertips can come up to your shins.

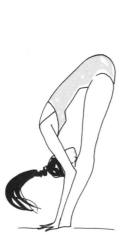
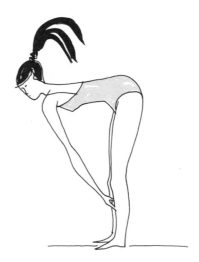

12. Mountain Pose: Exhale as you stand up, raising your arms to your sides in a slow, sweeping motion. End by bringing your hands up into prayer position at your heart center.

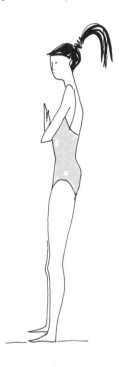

REPEAT THE SEQUENCE, this time stepping back with the left leg first. Keep repeating the entire sequence for 15 minutes.

13. Child's Pose: Always end your yoga flow by cooling down in Child's Pose. Sit back on your heels and then fold forward over your thighs and knees so your forehead touches the floor. Your arms are alongside your body, palms facing up. Hold the pose and breathe deeply for a few minutes.

14. *Savasana* (Corpse Pose): Now lie flat on your back, arms extended by your sides, palms facing up a short distance from your body. Your legs are slightly spread apart, heels heavy on the mat. Lie in this relaxing pose for at least 5 minutes to allow the energizing, revitalizing benefits of your practice to move through your body.

Sun Salutation: Intermediate

1. Mountain Pose: Stand with your feet together and parallel, big toes touching, and hands in front of your chest in prayer position. Your shoulder blades slide down your back, and your chin is parallel to the floor. Imagine pulling your navel to your spine. Take several deep breaths, inhaling and exhaling through your nose.

2. Hands Up: As you inhale, sweep your arms out to the sides and then up so they meet overhead. Gently arch your back, and look up toward your hands, making sure your abs are slightly contracted to avoid straining your lower back.

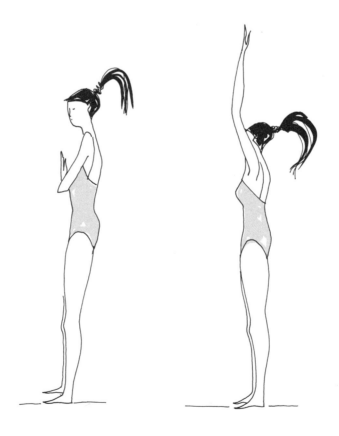

3. Forward Fold: On your next exhale, bend forward from the hinge of your hips, sweeping your arms straight out to the sides and then down so you can place your palms on the floor. Bend your knees if necessary.

4. Flat Back: Now inhale as you lift your head and direct your gaze forward, lengthening your spine. Your fingertips can come up to your shins.

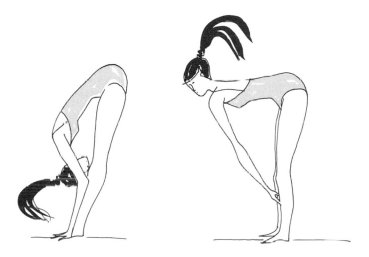

5. Forward Fold: Exhale and drop your head as you place your palms back on the floor, bending your knees if necessary.

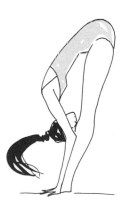

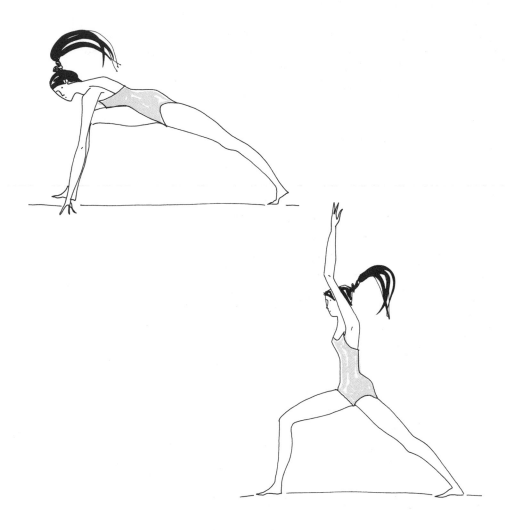

6. Lunge and Crescent Pose: Exhale and step your left foot back into a lunge position. Keep your right knee bent with your thigh parallel to the mat, and your left leg extended long behind you. Your hips and toes should face the front of your mat; your right foot is flat on the mat and your left toes curled under, so that your left heel is lifted. Now inhale and float your arms up and overhead, keeping them extended long and shoulder-width apart, with your palms facing each other. Exhale your hands back down to the mat, placing them on either side of your right foot.

7. Plank: Step the right foot back to meet the left and lower yourself into the Plank position. Your body should form a straight line from your head to heels, with your palms directly underneath your shoulders. The crown of your head reaches away from your toes, and your abdominals are engaged by pulling your navel up to your spine. Your toes are curled under. Hold the position and inhale.

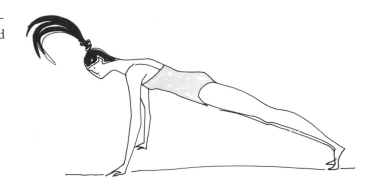

8. Stick: Exhale as you bend your elbows and lower yourself down, as if coming down from a push-up. Your elbows stay close to your sides, hugging your ribs, and your abdominals remain engaged by pulling your navel up to your spine. Only your hands and feet should touch the floor. If this is too strenuous, modify the pose by lowering yourself all the way down to the mat rather than hovering just above it.

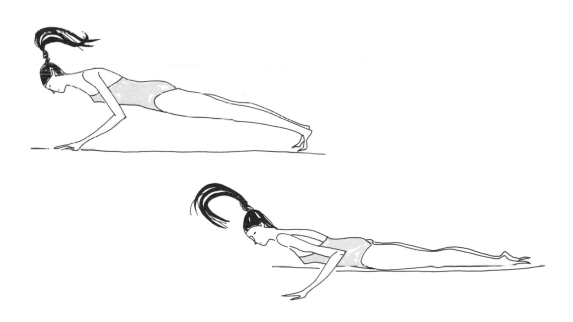

9. Upward-Facing Dog: Now inhale as you roll over your toes onto the tops of your feet, using your arms to push your chest forward and stretch your torso forward and up by bending at the waist. Bend your upper body back only as far as feels comfortable and safe, and never drop your head all the way back. Shoulders should be down and slightly rolled back. Only the tops of your feet and your hands should touch the floor. It's okay to keep your arms bent at the elbows.

10. Downward-Facing Dog: Now exhale as you press down with your palms and lift from the hips, rolling onto the balls of your feet and pushing back and up until your legs are straight. Your feet are hip-width apart, with your heels stretching down as close to the floor as possible and your hips reaching toward the sky. Lengthen your spine, and keep your hands shoulder-width apart. Or, take your gaze in toward your navel.

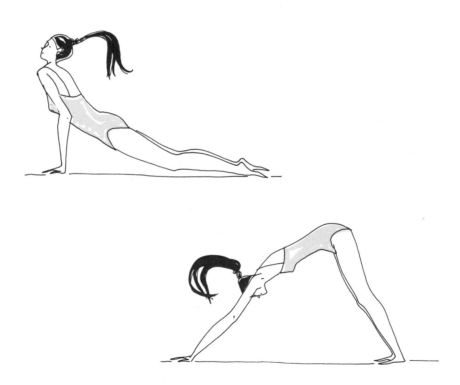

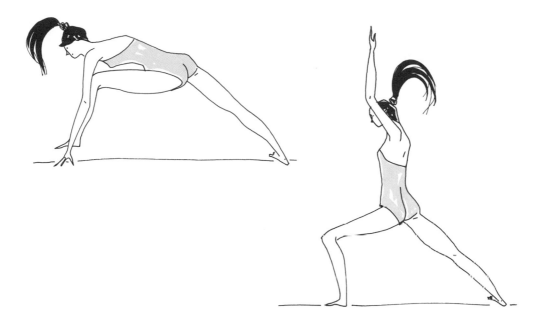

11. Lunge and Crescent Pose: Inhale as you step your left foot forward and place it between your hands so that you are in a lunge position. Your left thigh should be parallel to the mat, with your right leg extended and straight behind. Your hips and toes face the front of your mat. Your left foot is flat on the mat, and your right toes are curled under so that your right heel lifts from the mat. Now inhale and float your arms up and overhead, extended long, shoulder-width apart, palms facing each other.

12. Forward Fold: Exhale and bring your hands back down and place them on either side of your left foot. Inhale and bring your right foot forward to meet your left foot so your big toes are touching. Keep your palms on the floor and straighten your legs so that you are back in the Forward Fold position, your head at your knees.

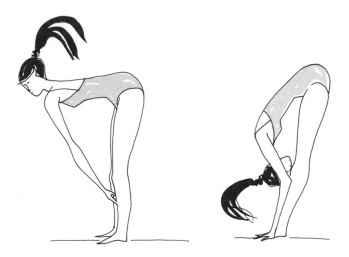

13. Flat Back: Inhale as you lift your head and direct your gaze forward to stretch and lengthen your spine. Your fingertips can come up to your shins.

14. Forward Fold: On your next exhale, drop your head as you place your palms back on the floor, bending your knees if necessary.

15. Mountain Pose: Exhale as you come up to standing and raise your arms out and up so your palms touch overhead. Then float your hands back down by your sides and bring them up into prayer position at your heart center.

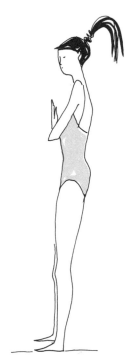

REPEAT THE SEQUENCE, this time stepping back with the right leg first. Keep repeating the entire sequence for 15 minutes.

16. Child's Pose: Again, always end your yoga flow by cooling down in Child's Pose. Sit back on your heels and then fold forward over your thighs and knees so your forehead touches the floor. Your arms are alongside your body, palms facing up. Hold the pose and breathe deeply for a few minutes.

17. *Savasana* **(Corpse Pose):** Now lie flat on your back, arms extended by your sides, palms facing up a short distance from your body. Your legs are slightly spread apart, heels heavy on the mat. Lie in this relaxing pose for at least 5 minutes to allow the energizing, revitalizing benefits of your practice to move through your body.

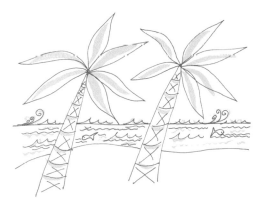

Sun Salutation: Advanced

1. Mountain Pose: Stand with your feet parallel and together, your big toes touching and your hands in front of your chest in prayer position. Slide your shoulder blades down your back, keeping your neck long and your chin parallel to the floor. Imagine pulling your navel back toward to your spine. Take several deep breaths, inhaling and exhaling through your nose.

2. Chair: Inhale as you bend your knees so that you are in a sitting position. Your arms are extended long by your sides, fingertips reaching toward the mat. With your knees still bent, float your arms up to the sides and then overhead, keeping them shoulder-width apart, with your palms facing toward one another and your upper inner arms close to your ears. Tuck your tailbone under to protect your lower back. Make sure your knees are directly over your toes.

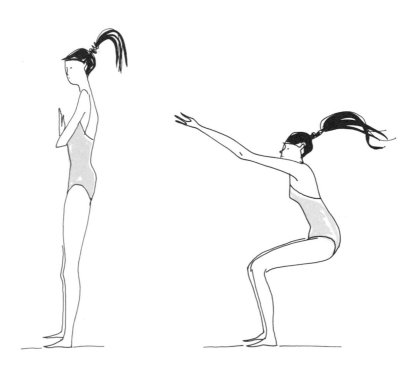

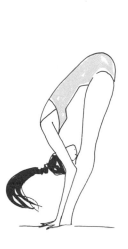
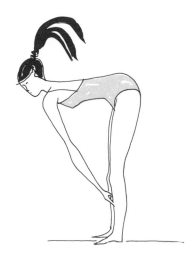

3. Forward Fold: On your next exhale, bend forward from the hinge of your hips, straighten your legs, and place your palms on the floor. Your knees can remain slightly bent if necessary.

4. Flat Back: Inhale as you lift your head and direct your gaze forward, extending and flattening your spine. Your fingertips can come up to your shins.

5. Forward Fold: Exhale and drop your head as you place your palms back on the floor, bending your knees if necessary.

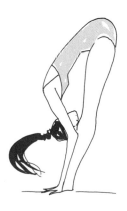

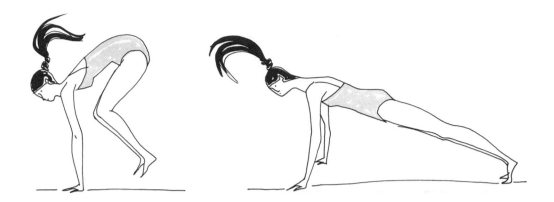

6. Plank: Inhale, bend your knees, and either step or jump back into Plank position. Your arms are straight and your body should form a straight line from your head to heels, with your palms directly underneath your shoulders, the crown of your head reaching away from your toes, and your abdominals engaged by pulling your navel up to your spine. Your toes are curled under.

7. Stick: Now exhale as you bend your elbows and lower yourself down as if coming down from a push-up. Your elbows stay close to your sides, hugging your ribs, and your abdominals remain engaged by pulling your navel up toward to your spine. Only your hands and feet should touch the floor.

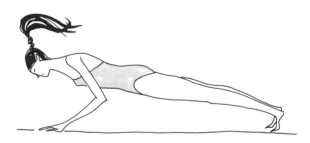

8. Upward-Facing Dog: Now inhale as you roll over your toes onto the tops of your feet, and use your arms to push your chest forward and stretch your torso forward and up, bending at the waist. Bend back only as far as feels comfortable and safe, and never let your head drop all the way back. Your shoulders should be down and slightly rolled back. Only the tops of your feet and your hands touch the floor. It's okay to keep your arms bent at the elbows.

9. Downward-Facing Dog: Exhale as you press down with your palms and lift from the hips, rolling onto the balls of your feet, and pushing back and up. Your feet are hip-width apart, with your heels stretching down toward the floor and your hips reaching toward the sky. Your hands are shoulder-width apart; your head is gazing downward or in toward your navel.

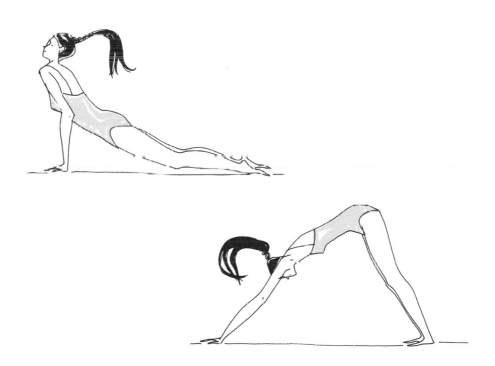

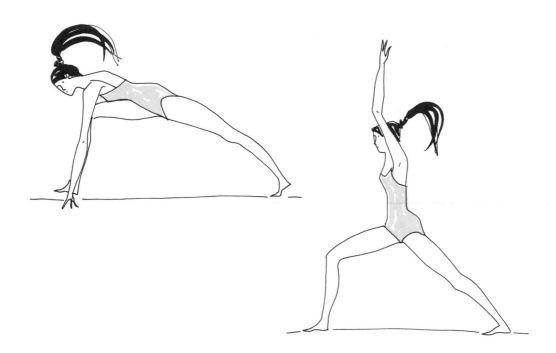

10. Warrior 1: Inhale and step your right foot forward into a lunge, pivoting your left heel 90 degrees outward so it is perpendicular to your body. Both feet are planted firmly on the floor and your right and left heels form a straight line with one another. Float your arms forward, up, and overhead, keeping them as straight as possible. Your hands are shoulder-width apart, with your palms facing each other and your fingers widespread. Both your hips should be rotated toward the front of your mat. Your right thigh should be parallel with the mat as you sink deeper into your lunge, never allowing your right knee to extend past your right toes. Your left leg is engaged and as straight as possible. Your weight should be evenly distributed over both legs, and your abdominals slightly contracted.

Bikini Tip

All yoga helps you manage stress more effectively, but these Warrior poses are particularly helpful in banishing butterflies from your stomach and building your confidence and energy before a crunch moment, say, a job interview or asking your boss for a raise.

11. Warrior 2: Exhale and lower your straight right arm down so it extends out in front of you, and your straight left arm down in back of you, so that they both come to shoulder height with the palms facing down. Keeping your feet and legs in the same position, rotate your hips and torso to the left so that you face the left side of your mat.

12. Reverse Warrior: From Warrior 2, inhale and slide your left hand down the back of your left thigh. At the same time, raise your right arm overhead, so it is in line with your right ear with the palm facing behind you. Your torso, neck, and head will automatically form a slight backbend. Your gaze is directed overhead.

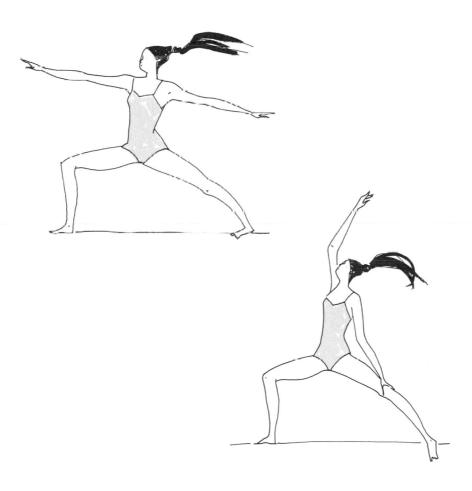

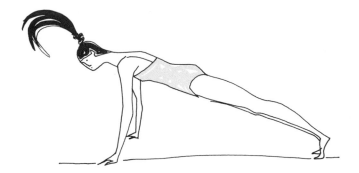

13. Plank: From Reverse Warrior, exhale and "cartwheel" your left arm forward so both arms come down in front of you and you can place both hands on either side of your right foot. Step your right leg back to meet your left leg and go into Plank position. Your head, neck, back, and legs form a straight line. Hold the position and inhale.

For the ultimate BBC experience, try doing Sun Salutations outside, on a porch, in a yard, or even in the park or on a nearby beach. As the name of the series indicates, it's a wonderful way to greet the sun and the natural world, and bring yourself into harmony with both.

14. Stick: Exhale as you bend your elbows and lower yourself down as if coming down from a push-up. Your elbows stay close to your sides, hugging your ribs, and your abdominals remain engaged by pulling your navel up toward your spine. Only your hands and feet should touch the floor.

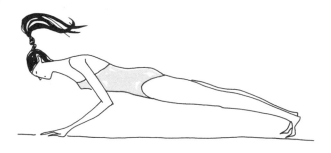

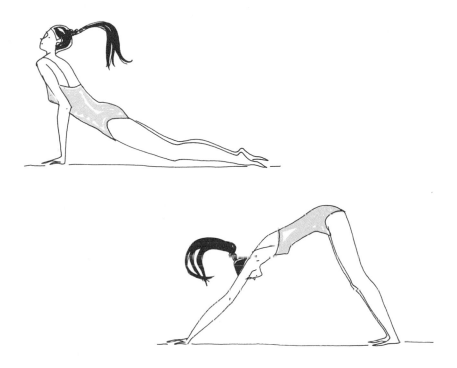

15. Upward-Facing Dog: Inhale as you roll over your toes onto the tops of your feet, and straighten your arms to push your chest forward, stretching your torso forward and up. Bend back only as far as feels comfortable and safe. Your shoulders should be relaxed down and slightly rolled back. Only the tops of your feet and your hands touch the floor. It's okay to keep your arms bent at the elbows.

16. Downward-Facing Dog: Now exhale as you press down with your palms and lift from the hips, rolling onto the balls of your feet and pushing back and up. Your feet are hip-width apart, your heels stretching toward the floor and your hips reaching toward the sky. Your hands are shoulder-width apart; your head is gazing down or in toward your navel.

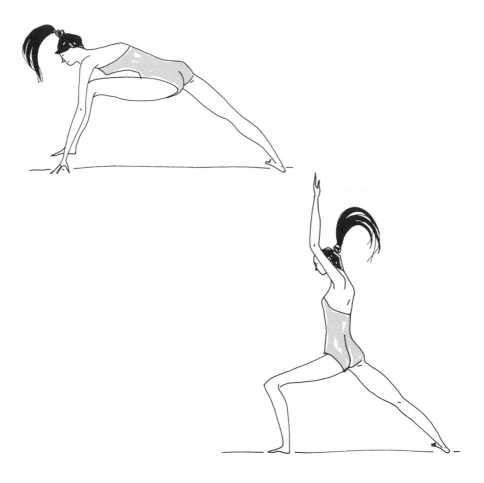

17. Warrior 1: Inhale and step your left foot forward into a lunge as you pivot your right heel 90 degrees outward so it is perpendicular to your body. Both feet are planted solidly on the floor, and your right and left heels form a straight line with one another. Now float your arms up and overhead, keeping them as straight as possible, with your hands shoulder-width apart and your palms facing each other, fingers widespread. Make sure your hips are rotated toward the front of your mat. Your left thigh is parallel with the mat as you sink deeper into your lunge, never allowing your left knee to extend past your toes. Your right leg is engaged and as straight as possible. Your weight should be evenly distributed between both legs and your abdomen slightly contracted.

18. Warrior 2: Exhale and lower your straight left arm so it extends out in front of you, and your straight right arm down in back, so that they both come to shoulder–height, with the palms facing down. Keeping your feet and legs in the same position, rotate your hips and torso to the right so that you face the right side of the mat.

19. Reverse Warrior: From Warrior 2, inhale and place your right hand on the back of your right thigh. As you slide your hand down your thigh, raise your left arm overhead so it is in line with your left ear, with the palm facing behind you. Your torso, neck, and head will automatically form a slight backbend. Your gaze is directed overhead.

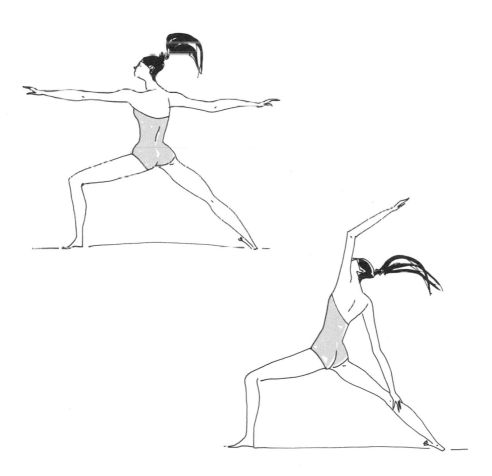

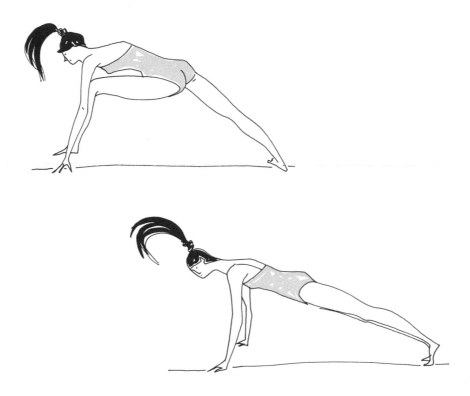

20. Plank: From Reverse Warrior, exhale and "cartwheel" your right arm forward so both arms come down in front of you and you can place both hands on either side of your left foot. Then step your left leg back to meet your right and go into Plank pose. Make sure your head, neck, back, and legs form a straight line. Hold the position and inhale.

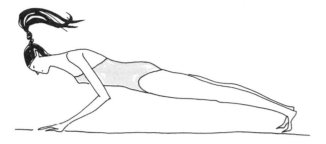

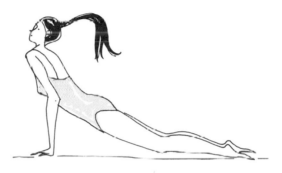

21. Stick: Exhale as you bend your elbows and lower yourself down as if coming down from a push-up. Your elbows stay close to your sides, hugging your ribs, and your abdominals remain engaged by pulling your navel up toward your spine. Only your hands and feet should touch the floor.

22. Upward-Facing Dog: Now inhale as you roll over your toes onto the tops of your feet, using your arms to push your chest forward, and stretching your torso forward and up by bending at the waist. Bend back only as far as feels comfortable and safe. Your shoulders should be down and slightly rolled back. Lift your legs up so that only the tops of your feet and your hands touch the floor. It's okay to keep your arms bent at the elbows.

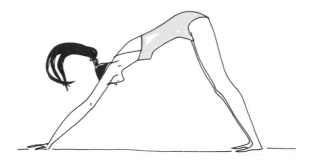

23. Downward-Facing Dog: Exhale as you press down with your palms and lift from the hips, rolling onto the balls of your feet, and pushing back and up. Your feet are hip-width apart, your heels stretch toward the floor, and your hips reach toward the sky. Your hands are shoulder-width apart; your head is gazing down or in toward your navel.

24. Forward Fold: Step or jump your feet forward to land in between your hands. Keeping your palms on the floor, straighten your legs to return to the Forward Fold position, your head at your knees.

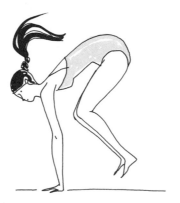
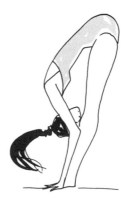

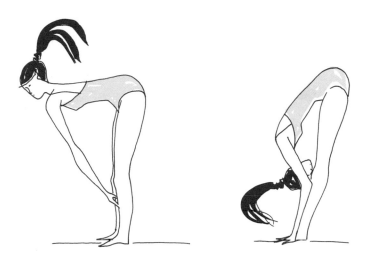

25. Flat Back: Inhale as you lift your head to gaze forward and lengthen your spine. Your fingertips can come up to your shins.

26. Forward Fold: Now exhale as you drop your head and place your palms back on the floor, bending your knees if necessary.

27. Chair: Inhale as you bend your knees and straighten your back so that you are in a sitting position. Your arms are extended long by your sides, fingertips pointing toward the mat. With your knees still bent, float your arms forward and overhead, keeping them shoulder-width apart, with the palms facing one another and your upper inner arms close to your ears. Tuck your tailbone under and contract your abs slightly to protect your lower back. Make sure your knees do not extend past your toes.

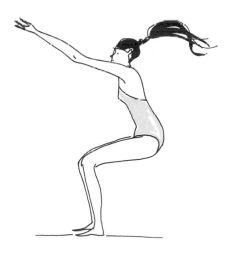

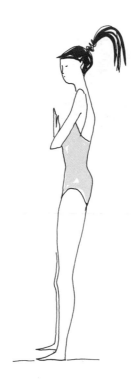

28. Mountain Pose: Now exhale as you come up to standing, raising your arms to let your palms touch overhead, and then floating them back down by your sides. End by bringing your hands up to prayer position at your heart center.

REPEAT THE SEQUENCE for 15 minutes.

29. Child's Pose: End your yoga flow by cooling down in Child's Pose. Sit back on your heels and then fold forward over your thighs and knees so your forehead touches the floor. Your arms are alongside your body, palms facing up. Hold the pose and breathe deeply for a few minutes.

30. *Savasana* **(Corpse Pose):** Now lie flat on your back, arms extended by your sides, palms facing up a short distance from your body. Your legs are slightly spread apart, heels heavy on the mat. Lie in this relaxing pose for at least 5 minutes to allow the energizing, revitalizing benefits of your practice to move through your body.

Additional Asanas

As you improve your yoga practice, you can try additional yoga postures that address your particular concerns: improving posture, abdominal strength, or even eliminating toxins. These postures are not a critical part of your flow sequence, but they are fun to do and they feel great. Just add them, as needed, to the mandatory flow routines.

CAT POSE FOLLOWED BY COW POSE

(for spinal release)

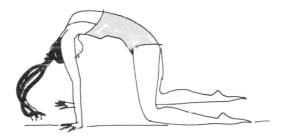

1. Position yourself on the mat on your hands and knees, wrists directly under your shoulders, knees hip-width apart and directly under your hips

2. Contract and lift your abs slightly so your spine and neck are relaxed, elongated, and curving slightly downward, with your chin slightly tucked in.

3. Inhale deeply and then exhale as you lift and curve your back upward, dropping your head down and curling your tailbone under.

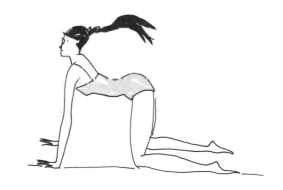

4. Now inhale as you reverse the spinal curve, lifting your tailbone, drawing your shoulders back, and raising your chest and head as far as you can as your spine softens and your abdominal muscles relax. You need to maintain a degree of contraction so your spine doesn't collapse totally. Repeat for 5 breath cycles.

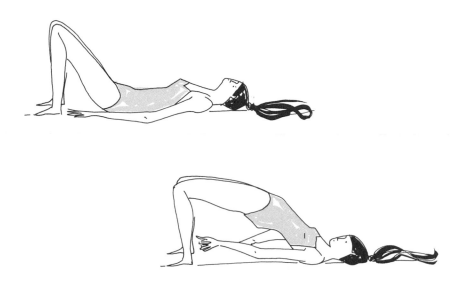

BRIDGE POSE (for spinal strength)

    1. Lie on your back and bend your knees, with your heels planted flat on the floor and about 6 inches from your hips. Your arms are extended on the floor alongside your torso, palms down.

    2. As you inhale, push down through your feet and lift your hips and torso up off the floor to form a straight line from your shoulders to your knees. Both hips should be squared to the ceiling and your knees should be lined up over your ankles. Now rock gently from side to side to fold your shoulders back underneath you as you bring your arms under your body and interlace your hands beneath your hips. Press your shoulders down and together to open your chest and relax your throat and jaw. Hold for 3 breaths and work up to 10 breaths.

BOAT POSE (abdominal strengthener)

1. Begin in a seated position, your back straight, your hands on the floor at your sides. Your knees are bent and touching, with your feet on the floor in front of you.

2. Lift your feet off the mat so that your shins are parallel to the floor. Keep your abs contracted and your back straight.

3. Now lift your hands off the floor, palms facing one another, and hold them at knee height. Hold for 5 breaths, maintaining the contraction in your abs throughout.

4. To make the Boat Pose even more challenging, straighten both legs and hold for 5 breaths.

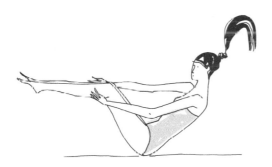

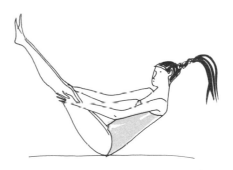

RECLINED TWIST POSE (for detoxifying)

1. Lie flat on your back on your mat. Inhale as you draw both knees into your chest and extend your arms out to your sides on the floor, at shoulder level.

2. Exhale as you drop your knees gently to the right and turn your head to the left, making sure both shoulders remain in contact with the floor. Let your weight sink into the floor as you relax, and breathe 3 times.

3. Inhale as you roll your knees back to center, and then exhale as you drop your knees to the left and roll your head to the right side. Hold for 3 breaths. Repeat each round 3 to 10 times.

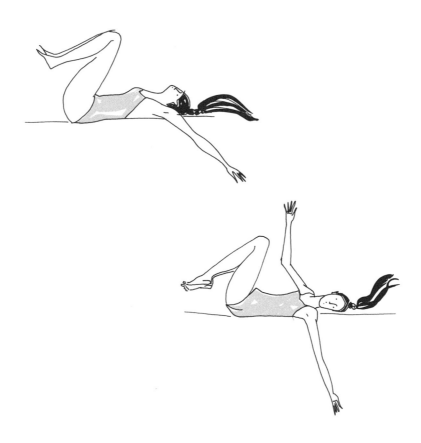

Yoga Practice Tips

- Yoga should ideally be done on a yoga mat—a six-foot or so length of thin rubber specially designed to prevent slipping and to cushion your body against the hard floor or ground. If you don't have a mat, a towel spread over a firm surface will work as well.
- Wear comfortable clothing that allows you to move easily from posture to posture. Do not wear shoes or socks.
- Although you need to do only 15 minutes of Vinyasa flow each day to see results, try to work up to 30 to 45 minutes of flow as you get stronger. The more you do, the greater that caloric burn.
- It's hard to do yoga on a full stomach, so if you can't do your Sun Salutations when you first wake up, leave at least one hour—two hours is ideal—between your last meal and the start of your practice.
- Do not let a lack of space inhibit your practice. All you need is space for your mat. If you can't reach your arms to the sides because there's not enough room (as may be the case for apartment dwellers), you can always hold your hands in prayer at your heart center or extend them out in front of you instead of extending your arms out to your sides.
- As you progress, challenge yourself by holding the postures longer, or by moving at a more rapid pace, increasing the duration of your practice, or adding in postures from a more advanced sequence.
- Even as you become familiar with the sequences and begin to pick up speed, always move slowly through the flow the first time to warm your muscles.
- Do not let yoga breathing intimidate you. Your awareness of your breath will build as you become more comfortable with your practice.
- As a general rule of thumb, long exhalations relax, while long inhalations give added energy. However, yoga experts advise that inhalations should never be longer than exhalations, as that can tax your heart. You'll find several other breathing exercises—or *pranayamas*—in the pages that follow, which you can practice anytime you need to calm down or reenergize.

Music to Flow By

Once you've mastered the poses and are able to synchronize your inhalations and exhalations to your movements, you may find that music with the right rhythm and tempo enhances the fluidity of your flow and removes you even further from the pressures and stresses of everyday life. Too slow and your practice will drag; too fast and you will feel frenetic and be tempted to speed up. So choose music that appeals to you, no matter what the genre, as long as it has a strong, steady beat and a medium tempo.

BIKINI BOOTCAMP MUSICAL FLOW FAVORITES
1. Bryan Ferry, "Avalon"
2. Dixie Chicks, "Landslide"
3. 10,000 Maniacs, "If You Intend"
4. Des'ree, "Life"
5. Delerium and Sarah McLachlan, "Silence"
6. Toto, "Africa"
7. James Blunt, "Beautiful Dawn"
8. Credence Clearwater Revival, "Have You Ever Seen the Rain"
9. Dire Straits, "Romeo and Juliet"
10. Cat Stevens, "Oh Very Young"
11. Deva Premal, "Om Mani Padme Hum"
12. Paris Lounge, "Llorac"

Pranayamas (Breathing Exercises)

Yoga breathing exercises—called *pranayamas*—are a great way to increase breath awareness and balance your energy, either calming or energizing you depending on your needs. As you experiment with these exercises, you want to focus your attention on how your body is reacting to the different breathing patterns in order to balance your needs for each day. Some people need to relax *before* they can tap into energy reserves they haven't been using; others need extra energy in order to get through challenging situations—including a tough new workout regimen.

Feel free to repeat favorites and not to practice others, always listening to your body and honoring what works best for you. We recommend

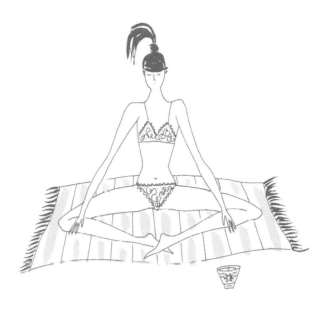

that you start with a relaxing breathing exercise, like Alternate Nostril Breathing, and if you find yourself falling asleep or bored out of your mind, kick in an energizing *pranayama,* like Breath of Fire. You can use these *pranayamas* throughout your BBC program either to unwind at the end of your workouts or, if you're feeling sluggish, to give youself a much-needed energy boost.

Alternate Nostril Breathing (to calm down)

The most basic *pranayama,* Alternate Nostril Breathing calms and clears the mind and strengthens respiratory function. After a long day of Bikini Bootcamp, it's a wonderful way to relax your tired body before going to sleep at night.

1. Sit on a chair or cross-legged with your eyes closed and press your thumb against your right nostril.
2. Inhale through your left nostril, counting up to 4.
3. Now press your ring finger against your left nostril as you release your thumb and slowly exhale through the right nostril to the count of 4 or more.
4. Inhale through the right nostril to the count of 4.

5. Release your ring finger from your left nostril, and press your thumb to close off the right nostril once again. Exhale through the left nostril to the count of 4 or more.

This constitutes one round; do at least 10 rounds for full calming and energizing effects. As you become more accustomed to the breath, try increasing the count of your inhalations and exhalations.

Prayer Breath (calms and relaxes)
1. Stand straight and tall, your feet hip-width apart and your palms together in front of your chest in prayer position. Your shoulders should be relaxed down and slightly pulled back.
2. Exhale as you sweep your arms out and down to your sides, and then inhale and bring them back to prayer position. Repeat 3 to 10 times, timing the movement of your arms to your inhalations and exhalations and making your exhalations slightly longer.
3. Now place your hands in prayer position and inhale as you bring your arms out by your sides, and then sweep them up so your palms touch overhead.
4. Exhale as you draw your pressed palms back down the center of your body, stopping in front of your heart. Repeat 3 to 10 times, making your exhalations longer and longer with each repetition.

Breath of Fire (clears and energizes the body and brain)
Whenever you need a jump-start, try this yogic breathing exercise. It's a great follow-up to your morning Sun Salutations because it wakes you up and gets you going far more effectively than a cup of coffee. Plus it's a great abs toner! You can do this *pranayama* while standing, sitting cross-legged, or seated in a chair, and you want to keep your eyes and your mouth closed.
1. Exhale forcefully through your nose as you sharply contract your abs, visualizing them touching your spine.
2. Now inhale. Allow the inhalation to come spontaneously through your nose, without ever forcing it. Your abs relax to allow breath to fill your body.
3. Repeat this pattern slowly, gradually building the speed of your abs contractions, without losing a steady, even rhythm. Start with 10 rounds (one exhalation and inhalation) and build from there.

Never do more than 50 rounds. If you begin to hyperventilate or feel dizzy, stop and allow your breath to return to normal.

4. Finish by bringing your right palm to your belly. Inhale deeply through your nose, filling your belly, and then exhale from your mouth with a deep, loud "aah" sigh. Lower both hands into your lap, palms facing up, and remain still for a few moments.

At the end of our yoga practice we say *"Namaste,"* which means "The divine, the light in me recognizes and honors the divine, the light in you." Even if you're practicing alone, why not say it and honor yourself?

CHAPTER 4

Walking

To resist the frigidity of old age, one must combine the body, the mind, and the heart—and to keep them in vigor, one must exercise, study, and love.
—*Karl von Bonstetten*

Walking is perhaps the world's easiest form of exercise—and it delivers great results! At Bikini Bootcamp, our guests and our dogs enjoy power walks on Tulum's long expanse of beach, where the sand ups the toning and endurance benefits as well as the calorie burn by 30 to 50 percent. If there's a beach near your area, you can replicate this challenging experience, but if you have back problems, walking on sand involves constant shifting, so you're better off on a flat, stable surface. In any case, wherever you walk, once you're doing it properly, this wonderfully simple exercise is just as effective as more strenuous aerobic activities. It promotes weight loss by increasing your metabolism and improves muscle tone while putting far less stress on your knees and joints than running. Best of all, there's no need for a personal trainer or special equipment—just comfortable clothes and supportive walking shoes or sneakers.

The right shoes should suit both your feet and your specific walking terrain. A specialty shoe store, podiatrist, or sports medicine doctor can help, especially if you tend to overpronate (roll your feet inward), supinate (roll outward if your arches are overly high), or even if you just walk normally and want the best support. For a perfect fit, try on walking shoes after you've exercised and your feet are a bit swollen from the activity. Your shoe should be half an inch longer than the length of your longest toe. We recommend wearing merino wool or synthetic blend socks to prevent blisters, and avoiding cotton because it traps sweat.

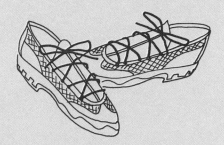

Your daily walk—anywhere from thirty minutes to an hour, depending on your fitness level—will probably be the easiest part of your Bikini Bootcamp program. After all, most of us already do some form of walking every day. There are no postures to learn or circuits to master; nevertheless, there is a right way to walk if you really want to see results.

Always hold your body tall, stretching from the bottom of your spine to the top of your head, your neck and chin slightly tucked, your chest slightly out, your shoulders down and slightly rolled back. Your feet should be parallel, toes pointing straight ahead. You want to sense your core muscles and tighten them just a bit. This posture protects your back and ensures that your entire body is working efficiently.

- Find your stride length by standing with your feet together. Lean forward from your ankles until you are forced to take a step. Wherever your heel lands is your proper stride length when walking for fitness.
- Hit the ground heel first and roll through your foot, pushing off with your toes. This motion also helps your leg muscles move blood to your heart so it doesn't overwork.
- Start by walking for five minutes at an easy warm-up pace. Then take faster steps to burn more calories and get your heart rate up. Your target heart rate should be between 65 and 80 percent of your maximum heart rate (see "Finding Your Target Heart Rate" below).
- Bend your elbows at a 90-degree angle and move your arms in a controlled way in time with your feet. Cup your hands loosely. Avoid moving your arms in an uncontrolled fashion as this can cause tendinitis (inflammation of the connective tissue).
- Look straight ahead, glancing down from time to time to scan the terrain.

- Take five minutes to cool down after your walk by slowing your pace and continuing to move until your pulse reaches below 65 percent of your maximum heart rate. This avoids sudden muscle contractions that can cause your blood pressure to drop too sharply.
- After your cooldown, finish off with a Downward-Facing Dog posture (see page 77) to stretch your muscles.

How Long Should You Walk?

The optimal duration of your walk is one hour—but depending on your current fitness level, you may need to start off walking for shorter intervals and build up. No matter how long you walk, you want to be sure to move at a pace that challenges you. Walking at a brisk pace, you'll cover about two miles every half hour. Your ultimate goal should be roughly 10,000 steps, or five miles, a day. In the meantime, here's how to find your start point for the BBC program.

If you haven't been exercising regularly: Start out with 30 minutes of brisk walking and increase the duration every four days as outlined in the daily plans in Part II. By Day 10 you should be walking the full hour, even if you have to slow down from time to time.

If you have been exercising regularly: Aim for the full hour power walk from the start. If walking comes easy and you're looking for an extra challenge, try increasing the caloric burn by wearing a weighted vest, trying out some hilly terrain, or, if you walk on a treadmill, programming some more challenging intervals into the mix. Never carry weights in your hands or strapped to your ankles, as this increases your risk of injury or muscle strain.

Finding Your Target Heart Rate

In order to derive the maximum bikini benefits from your walks, it's important to know your target heart rate. Tracking your heart rate, or pulse, while you exercise allows you to measure exactly how hard your body's working and ensure that the pace is challenging enough to zap away any extra pounds.

Your target heart rate is 65 to 80 percent of your maximum heart rate—that is, the fastest and hardest your heart can pump. To find your maximum heart rate, simply subtract your current age from 220. The number you are left with is your maximum heart rate; your target heart rate will be 65 to 80 percent of that. For example, if you're thirty years old, your maximum heart rate will be 190 and your target heart rate will be anywhere from 123 to 152 beats per minute. When you work out at this pace, 50 percent of the calories you are burning come from fat! So it's worth it to know your target numbers and make sure you stay in the zone throughout your walk.

To check your pulse, place your fingertips on the inside of your wrist right where it meets your hand. Count the number of beats for 15 seconds and then multiply that number by four.

Walking versus Running

In terms of burning calories, running for three miles burns more calories per minute. But walking for three miles—though it may take longer—burns the same amount of calories. Of course, walking is easier on the joints, and most people find it easier to incorporate into their daily lives than running. Furthermore, studies also show that walkers tend to keep off more of the weight they lose than runners.

Tips to Keep You Moving

- If your schedule allows, try to do your walking first thing in the morning or in the evening, either before or after dinner. If this is impossible, as it is for many women with children and jam-packed lives, it's okay to split your walk into two 30-minute segments, as long as you move at a pace that makes you work.
- One way to make sure you are hitting the correct range (a pulse rate of 65 to 80 percent of your maximum heart rate) is to walk with a friend and talk as you walk. If you're breathing somewhat hard but can still talk, you're in the target range. If you can't form complete sentences, you're exercising too hard.
- Find a walking buddy. The buddy system makes daily walking easier, as getting up and out the door is less of a chore when you know someone else is waiting for you. While you may not be able to gather up fifteen or so buddies like we do at BBC, find someone who lives nearby or make friends with other walkers in your community.

....

If you want to walk before dinner but feel too tired, try a blood sugar-stabilizing pick-me-up snack that contains protein, healthy fat, and carbs, like 11/2 teaspoons of natural peanut butter and 1 teaspoon of sugar-free jam on a slice of whole grain bread or rice cake; peanut or almond butter on an apple slice or piece of banana; low-fat yogurt with a few slices of banana; or low-fat Wheat Thins or Triscuits with hummus or a thumb-size piece of low-fat cheese. See our list of healthy snacks on page 194 for other ideas.

- Use your newfound knowledge of yogic breathing to combine meditation with your walk. Focus on breathing in to the count of three and exhaling to the count of three, keeping your breathing even and regular. Or listen to a CD of chanting.
- Mix it up! Change your speed from a brisk pace to an even faster speed every five minutes to keep from getting bored. This type of interval training will also help you burn more calories.
- Another boredom-buster is to switch the location of your walk every so often or vary your route to keep your walks novel and fun. If you normally walk around the block, drive to a nature preserve for a change in scenery. Don't be afraid to add some hills to up the caloric burn even more.
- Check your community for charity race walks, especially those events that also offer pre-race training. Walking with others is a great way to make sure you stay motivated.
- The most important thing is to *just do it*. Don't sabotage your program by delaying getting out of the house! For each minute you delay, the chances that you will take your walk decrease dramatically. Someone will call; you'll notice a picture that needs dusting or an eyebrow that need plucking. Just go.

Walking Extras

We hope that these next fourteen days will inspire you to make walking a part of your life for good. And once you're committed to using walking for fitness, there are a few pieces of equipment that can make tracking your progress that much easier. If you have trouble finding your pulse or don't want to have to bother with counting and calculations during your workout, you can purchase a **heart rate monitor** for less than a hundred dollars. There's no better way to ensure that your walks are getting the job done.

A **pedometer** can also help you keep moving throughout your day by showing the distance you cover. Select a model that tracks only steps, as more complicated ones tend to be inaccurate. Clip the pedometer to your waistband or belt, directly over your right or left hipbone, and wear it from the time you get dressed in the morning until you go to bed at night. Jot down your step count each day and log your activities. Each week, total your numbers and make a list of what helps you and what hinders you. For example, if you're running an errand or driving to work, park several blocks from your destination to squeeze in more steps. Remember, you should be aiming for the BBC goal of 10,000 steps per day (about five miles).

A study in the *New England Journal of Medicine* conducted in 2003 found that just two and a half hours of brisk walking a week can cut your risk of heart attacks and strokes by nearly one-third because walking raises your levels of HDL (good) cholesterol and lowers blood pressure. Five hours of brisk walking per week does you even more good by cutting your risk of heart disease in half! You may be years away from worrying about these issues, but it's good to know that you're cultivating a habit that promises a long, healthy life.

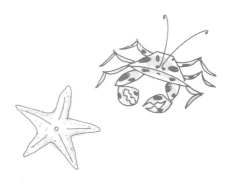

CHAPTER 5

Bikini Body Fuel

From the sky, from the earth, from a scrap of paper,
from a passing shape, from a spider's web . . . we must pick out
what is good for us where we can find it.
—*Pablo Picasso*

You wouldn't even be reading this book if you didn't already know that how you eat affects how you feel and look. When it comes to your health and appearance, the old maxim "You are what you eat" couldn't be truer. What's more, it stays true throughout your lifetime. So, the word *diet* does not exist in the Bikini Bootcamp vocabulary. After all, who wants to be on a diet for the next fifty years?

There is a Bikini Bootcamp *Lifestyle,* however, and healthy, enjoyable eating is key to our way of losing weight and keeping it off. Whether it's sugar-phobic, carb-busting, fat-avoiding, or meat-centric, "diet" implies restricting amounts and types of food. Diets are about desire and denial, and that's no fun. You've already learned that you can tone your Bikini Bootcamp body while enjoying yourself, and that includes shedding un-wanted pounds. Let's face it: You can't discipline yourself out of your nat-ural desire for food. So if you think losing weight is a matter of willpower, you are destined to fail.

Our secret to shedding pounds and keeping them off for the rest of your life is not compulsive dieting, but eating nutritious, low-calorie, high-fiber, *back-to-basics* foods like fruits, vegetables, lean proteins, and a few whole grains instead of high-calorie and unhealthy processed foods like white breads, fast foods, and sweets that pack on pounds and ruin your health. Those foods can wreak havoc with your blood sugar and leave you

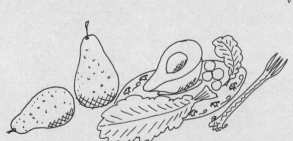

feeling depleted and sedentary rather than energized. In other words, sticky buns give you sticky buns!

The Bikini Body eating plan is a delicious and healthy way of fueling your body to give you maximum energy, glowing skin, *and* the best part—thinner thighs, hips, arms, and everything else. Our low-cal meals work in tandem with your workouts to decrease your calorie intake, boost your energy, keep your metabolism supercharged, and radically increase the number of calories you burn each day. That's a recipe for weight loss! In less than one week you will start to notice your pants fitting looser around your middle and your energy levels rising. You can expect to lose *at least* three pounds the first week simply by following the program for each day. By the end of two weeks you will have lost anywhere from four to ten pounds, depending on your starting weight and fitness level. Keep in mind that muscle weighs more than fat, so if the numbers on the scale don't drop as dramatically as you'd like, it's likely because you're firming up and building muscles in places you've never had them before!

We hope that the dishes you'll enjoy in Part II won't remind you of "health food," or "diet food," or even "spa food" in any way. At Bikini Bootcamp headquarters we serve this food to everyone, not only to those people wanting to lose weight—and they all inevitably come to us asking for the recipes. In fact, you can serve any of the meals here to guests, and they will never suspect that they are part of a weight-loss program.

The recipes embody our back-to-basics philosophy by emphasizing foods that are close to their natural state and eliminating foods that are processed and therefore no longer as fresh and nutritious as they should be. Eating this way supplies your body with the fuel it needs: lean protein in the form of grilled fish or chicken helps you build muscle and keeps your metabolism revved throughout the day; increased fiber through tasty chickpeas, spinach salads, and Mexican jicama helps your body cleanse itself of toxins and gives you a feeling of satiety so that you never feel deprived; healthy fats from nuts and avocados help you absorb essential nutrients and keep your skin radiant and smooth; and the antioxidants found in mangoes, pineapples, bananas, tomatoes, and other delicious fruits and vegetables boost your immune system and keep your body functioning in high gear.

Farmers' markets have become increasingly popular and can now be found in most major cities. Make an hour at your local farmers' market part of your weekend ritual so you can stock up on foods for the week ahead—it's a great way to ensure that whatever you're eating travels directly from the earth to your plate. Ethnic markets also offer an amazing array of exotic produce that can add variety to your menus.

⋯⋯

As you become more familiar with the Bikini Bootcamp way of eating, you will know right away whether a food is back-to-basics and good for you or refined and bad for you. The general rule of thumb is that you should stick to foods that have no more than one step between their sources and your plates. That means avoiding processed foods and beverages (those that are canned, packaged, and loaded with extra sugar and additives designed to enhance flavor and give the products a long shelf life); saturated fats that make bodies feel heavy and tired; and hormone-laced meats that put unwanted chemicals into your bloodstream. You will see that you can create delicious meals without frying, refined flour, white sugar, red meat, cream, or chemicals. The best part of it all is that the less the food is tampered with, the easier and faster it is to prepare.

Bear in mind that this new way of eating will be an adjustment for your body. It's like changing the gasoline you put in your car. How your body will react to being cut off from refined carbs and sugars, red meat, and bad fats depends on what your system is used to. You may initially experience sugar cravings or a yearning for fatty foods. Many of you will also undergo a dramatic increase in your fiber intake, which may make you feel bloated during the first few days—but this is not weight gain, nor is it permanent. These responses are normal and will quickly subside. It can take anywhere from three to five days to break your body into this new way of eating, but stick with it! Your belly will soon flatten and your energy levels will soar. In fact, most of our campers find that by the time they leave, they have actually lost their taste for sugar and fatty foods—something they never imagined could be possible.

Simply thinking about your food in this way will transform you into what we call a "focused" eater who respects and savors the food that nurtures her. Most people rarely give their relationship to food much attention, which is often what leads to weight gain and unhealthy habits. Unfocused eaters shove food into their mouths on automatic pilot, often utterly unaware of what they are putting into their system. They reach for whatever is convenient and available; they eat meals standing up in the kitchen or while watching TV or talking on the phone; and they usually have no idea of what or how much they've just consumed.

If you've been an unfocused eater in the past, all that will change once you begin eating the Bikini Bootcamp way. You will begin to desire foods that are closer to their natural and unadulterated state, and you'll see first-hand that this type of food makes you feel fabulous and won't pack on the pounds. Many people on our program feel as though their entire body "wakes up," so great is their newfound vigor and clarity. You'll taste food fully as it enters your mouth and savor the flavors as you take enough time to chew it well for healthier digestion. Best of all, the foods you come to crave will be the same ones that are good for your body, and you'll never have to think about dieting again.

Are You Really Hungry?

Part of committing to losing weight means learning to think about hunger in a whole new light. Most of us, at least some of the time, reach for food as a result of something other than true physical need. We eat to be so-cial—at parties, at business lunches, at gatherings with friends. We eat from boredom, when we're waiting for the cable guy to arrive and find ourselves snacking in the kitchen to pass the time. We eat to avoid letting food go to waste—we can't tell you the number of BBC moms who swear that at home they end up finishing their children's meals, even after they've had their own! And all too often, we eat to squelch difficult emotions: hurt feelings, anger, loneliness, and stress.

Part of changing your eating habits for the long-haul involves learning to eat *only* when your body is truly hungry, and not when outside circumstances urge you to reach for potato chips or a bowl of ice cream. One easy way to pinpoint any unhealthy reasons why you're eating is to keep a temporary food diary. Although your Bikini Bootcamp journal (more about this in Chapter 6) is intended primarily as a place to record your aspirations, hopes, and successes throughout these weeks rather than a place to count calories, if you have been having serious problems with overeating or bingeing—or even if you're simply curious to know where your calories are coming from—we recommend giving the food diary a try.

Here's how it works: Anytime you eat, write down how you feel before you begin eating, and then document what you ate, how much, and how you felt afterward. Be as honest with yourself as possible. You want to do this not only for the planned BBC meals, but for any little extras that you succumb to along the way—a cookie at an office party, a spontaneous latte when you're running errands (that Starbucks coffee aroma just smells so *good*!). Not only will this provide a record of how and when you eat, and where the extra calories might be sneaking in, but it also serves to highlight any emotional triggers that factor into your relationship with food. You will soon recognize patterns in your eating habits. Were you happy and energized, tired and lethargic, or uncomfortable and irritable before and after eating? Did you reach for the Ben & Jerry's after a phone call with your mother, or after bumping into your ex and his attractive female friend? After a few days you'll have a much clearer picture of your eating patterns and will be able to take action to stop unfocused eating before it starts. Doing so will greatly improve your chances of keeping the weight off after these two weeks are up—and going forward, you'll no longer feed your stomach when you really need to feed your soul.

Keep a List of "Craving Distractions"

If you typically experience cravings, it's a good idea to formulate a plan for dealing with them before you start the BBC program. In your journal, list at least fifteen activities you can do instead whenever you have an urge to eat that is not based on hunger or in compliance with the plan. Walk the dog, phone a friend, do your nails, or work on a fun, do-it-yourself project. One camper we know made all her wedding invitations by hand while undergoing an at-home version of our regimen before her big day. Remember to also use your new tools: yoga, walking, *pranayamas,* and the other workouts to keep you out of the kitchen when you should be on the move.

The Bikini Bootcamp Meal Plans

The meal plans we have created for you are built around the same culinary treats we serve to our guests at the spa. The recipes incorporate the best elements of the Mexican diet (fresh tropical fruit, fresh fish, vegetables, black beans, tomatoes, and avocados) and often combine them with Asian flavors for simple, delicious, nutritious eating. All the meals are low-cal, high in fiber, balanced in protein, full of vitamins, minerals, and antioxidants, and packed with lots of tasty zip thanks to a variety of spices. We use a few whole-grain carbs, such as amaranth (a grain indigenous to Mexico that's available here in the United States), soba noodles (buckwheat), and couscous (whole wheat, if available in your area). We're also not afraid of using healthy fats, such as those found in avocados and olive oil, as well as nuts and seeds, as they won't clog your arteries or pack on pounds and they are essential for your body to be able to process all of the nutrients in your new eating plan. We want you to enjoy your meals more than you ever have before. After all, the Bikini Bootcamp credo is to make it fun!

Before you start the program, we recommend that you eliminate from your kitchen all packaged, oversalted, trans-fat-laden, and non-nutritive food. You will likely find this purge liberating and be delighted to discover that it's much easier than you believed to prepare your own healthy dishes. Keep in mind, however, that you never want to eliminate any food group in its entirety! Every now and then we get guests at Bikini Bootcamp who announce that they want to undergo an even more restricted diet than what we offer. They say, "I don't want *any* fruit while I'm here because I don't want *any* carbs," or, "No guacamole for me; I want to eat completely fat-free this week." But please listen to us when we say that you need *all* the food groups you'll find in the recipes in order to complete the program successfully. You're going to be burning more energy than ever before, so you absolutely need some fats and carbs, and you need protein as well to help repair and build muscle tissue after your workouts. This is not another fad diet built solely around grapefruit or cabbage or red meat, and depriving yourself of any component of the program will only deplete your body rather than restore it to its healthy, radiant self.

In Mexico it's a breeze to use fresh, local ingredients, but we realize that this may be impractical for many readers to follow on a long-term basis. So we've provided you with a food plan that reflects our back-to-basics philosophy, but also makes some practical accommodations. The recipes are clear and precise; even if you are a cooking novice, you will have no problem following them, and you are free to interchange the meals in Part III for endless variety.

How It Works

At Bikini Bootcamp, we enjoy four meals a day: breakfast, lunch, an afternoon snack, and dinner accompanied by a soup to start and a dessert. You'll be eating lean protein at every meal, at least seven servings of fruits and vegetables, and more than 23 grams of fiber. If that sounds like a lot of food, it is! Remember, part of the BBC philosophy is never feeling deprived. But because even our desserts are deliciously low-cal, you'll still see the pounds disappear.

Breakfast

You may be one of those busy people who skips breakfast, settling instead for a cup of coffee sipped in your car or on the bus. If so, you are setting yourself up for hard-to-resist food cravings later in the day. You'll be so hungry by eleven o'clock that you can easily overeat at lunch, which will lead to a late-afternoon sugar crash and the temptation to gobble down a candy bar. By the time you get home you'll be ready to raid the fridge.

On the other hand, eating a healthy breakfast, such as those listed in Part II, will keep your blood sugar and appetite under control and your metabolism revved throughout the day. In fact, studies show that eating breakfast not only helps you lose weight, it also helps maintain weight loss. Many of our Bikini Bootcamp guests are surprised to discover that breakfast ends up being their favorite meal!

Lunch

Lunch at Bikini Bootcamp is always a salad, often full of fresh leafy greens, other veggies, and some form of protein, usually fish or chicken. Salads provide a hefty dose of fiber as well as key vitamins and minerals, and the variety of textures encourages you to chew longer and thus feel more satisfied. As you'll see, a salad does not have to contain lettuce, and many of our salads include beans, cabbage, spinach, and other fresh vegetables as their base. Our Amansala Salad with Ginger-Sesame Dressing is hands-down the most requested, most popular dish at BBC, and you'll enjoy it several times throughout the program. We guarantee you'll see why it gets raves from campers across the board!

When we make a salad at Amansala, we don't just pour on store-bought salad dressing, because even the vinaigrettes are laden with chemical preservatives, high-fructose corn syrup, fillers, and MSG. Instead, you'll be using our recipes for delectable, healthy, low-cal yet flavorful salad dressings that you can whip up in about two minutes. Keep them mixed and in your fridge for easy access whenever you're in a rush.

A Word about Dairy

As you review the meal plans, you'll likely notice that many of our breakfasts include low-fat yogurt. Dairy is a strong source of calcium, and research shows that by eating just two servings a day, whether in the form of low-fat cheese, milk, or yogurt, women can prevent osteoporosis and bone density loss as they get older. Mounting evidence also suggests that calcium may play a role in regulating body fat; a recent study of young women found that those who have low-fat yogurt or low-fat milk three times a week are less likely to gain weight. We're also fans of yogurt because each serving contains eight grams of protein—a great early-morning kick-start for your metabolism.

If you can't eat dairy, or really just don't like yogurt, you can substitute soy, nonfat, or lactose-free milk in any of the breakfast recipes in Part III. When it comes to snacks, you can choose an alternate from the complete list of healthy snacks on page 194).

Snacks

Snacks are an integral part of the Bikini Bootcamp lifestyle, and they keep your metabolism chugging throughout the day. The timing of your snack will differ for each of you, depending on when you usually eat lunch and when your blood sugar drops and you need an energy boost, though you should try to eat your snack *before* you feel hungry if you can. Your daily meal plan includes one snack each day, but if you're really dragging or need a pick-me-up prior to your afternoon workout, feel free to reach for any of the other healthy snacks listed in Part III (see page 194).

When choosing the snacks that suit your fancy, try to tailor your selections to your usual cravings. If you tend to crave something savory, eat a few whole-grain crackers or apple slices with peanut butter. Or replace salty potato chips with air-popped popcorn seasoned with chili and salt substitute, or quick-cook some edamame (fresh soybeans). If you crave sweets, replace Reese's Pieces with berries, watermelon, or frozen grapes. You can even substitute raisins for jelly beans.

Dinner

Dinner always starts with a yummy, low-cal vegetable soup, and if you've never made soup from scratch before, you'll be amazed at what a few vegetables and a blender can produce. Soups are a great, tasty source of nutrients and energy, and they fill you up so you're less inclined to overindulge in the main course or hanker for a late-night snack. They offer a creative way to get even more fresh vegetables into your diet, and the warmth gives us the sensation of comfort food—without any hidden fat!

We recognize that many of you are juggling busy schedules, so we recommend that you choose a few of the soups you like, make them in advance, and portion them out throughout the week so you don't have to make them every night. One serving of one soup is as good as another.

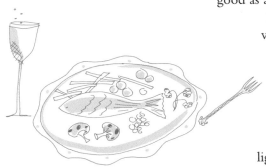

For the main course you'll enjoy a variety of options—from grilled shrimp to chicken fajitas to scrumptious fish tacos with our own Salsa Verde. We have also included a healthy dessert at the end of each meal. Dessert is the one part of the Bikini Bootcamp meal plan that is optional, so do not feel obligated to indulge. Only eat it if your sweet tooth really needs a fix, or if you are still feeling hungry or unsatisfied.

What to Drink

In Mexico we offer our campers plenty of water and herbal tea round the clock as well as a few signature beverages that you'll find in Part III. Staying hydrated is essential to your success at BBC, as you will feel less fatigued and therefore less tempted to give in to cravings for refined carbs and sugar. You'll want to aim for at least eight 8-ounce glasses of water or herbal tea a day; sugary drinks like sodas (including diet) and even all-natural fruit juices are strictly out because of the calorie count.

We also recommend something called a "Morning Burst"—a cup of hot water with a slice of fresh lemon that you enjoy when you wake up in the morning. Ideally, this should be the first thing to pass your lips. The lemon acts as a detoxifier, cleansing your system and readying you for the day.

If you can't make it out the door without your morning cup of coffee, or are used to drinking caffeinated teas, you can still enjoy these in the morning—so long as you avoid sugar and stick to a splash of low-fat milk. We would prefer that you avoid caffeine altogether, but we also recognize that trying to kick a lifelong coffee habit while taking on a strenuous exercise regimen and revamping your diet from top to bottom is a lot to ask. If you absolutely cannot stand your coffee unsweetened, you may add a touch of honey or an all-natural sweetener like stevia. Be careful with the honey, though—if you use it to sweeten eight cups of tea a day, the calories will add up quickly. So use it sparingly and try to opt for plain tea or coffee wherever possible.

And for all the girls about town who, like us, love a margarita or a martini now and then, for these two weeks alone—no booze! These empty calories will not satisfy your hunger, but they do add up. So put happy hour on hold until you have something great to celebrate: your newly toned and trimmed bikini body.

How to Eat

Over the next fourteen days, *how* you eat is just as important as *what* you eat. We instruct our campers on BBC meal etiquette on their very first night at dinner. The same goes for you! In order to get the most out the meal plan, follow these simple rules:

• **Don't skip meals.** You may save calories but you risk getting shaky and irritable and overeating later on. Remember, you'll already be cutting calories in a fairly significant way. Never skip breakfast—fruit with a bit of fat and protein is essential to keep your metabolism working properly. Having breakfast soon after you wake up kicks your metabolism into high gear.

- **It only takes a fist-size portion of food to appease your hunger.** This is your new mantra. Keep it in mind whenever you crave a snack. If you're hungry, it's okay to reach for something to nibble on; just make sure it comes from our approved snack list and doesn't turn into a full meal.

- **When eating, be fully present.** Do not eat while arguing, having serious discussions, or talking on the phone. Do not watch TV while eating, especially because of those snack food ads! If you are distracted or upset, set your meal aside, recenter yourself, and start eating again only when you are ready to focus on the food.

- **Eat slowly, taking your time to enjoy your meal.** Chew each bite of food thoroughly to enhance digestion. Remember, digestion starts in the mouth as necessary enzymes in your saliva mix with your food before it is sent down to your stomach. Eating more slowly ensures that you digest your food fully so your body can draw maximum benefits.

- **Make the ritual of eating a pleasure.** The food shouldn't be the only thing that draws you to the table. Even if you're eating alone, you can make your mealtimes more enjoyable by setting a place with beautiful tableware or linens, eating breakfast outdoors in the morning sun, lighting candles on your table in the evening, or taking a moment to express gratitude before you begin.

- **Stay hydrated.** Remember, at least eight 8-ounce glasses of water a day! Drinking plenty of water will help you feel less fatigued and flush any toxins from your workouts out of your system. Keep a one-liter bottle with you at all times and refill it as the day goes by.

- **Get enough zzzz's.** When you're tired, you're more likely to overeat, relying on caffeine, sugar, and refined carbs for an energy buzz. If you tend to make late-night fridge raids, try going to bed early instead.

- **"Failure" is not in the BBC vocabulary.** If you slip and inhale a bag of potato chips, don't beat yourself up and throw in the towel. You didn't fail; this process is ongoing. Simply go back to your back-to-basics eating at the next meal. In meditation, whenever we lose focus, we say, "Begin again." The same is true for the Bikini Bootcamp program.

Bikini Tip

Eat the best food you can afford. The quality of the calories you put into your mouth counts, so always opt for the freshest ingredients and choose organic wherever possible, whether you're buying yogurt, chicken breasts, or a head of lettuce. If you must buy something preprepared, frozen is better than canned or packaged any day.

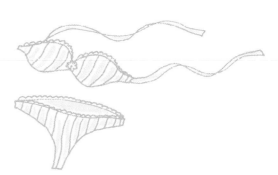

CHAPTER 6

The Bikini Body Mind-set

A ruffled mind makes a restless pillow.
—*Charlotte Brontë*

Sometimes it's not what you do but your approach to it that makes all the difference. As we've already told you, the Bikini Bootcamp program is not just for the body—it trains your mind and spirit as well, so you not only get the body you've always wanted, you get to keep it. By now you've learned all about the meal plans and the workouts, and you're probably itching to dive right in. But this chapter gives you essential information that will enable you to stay the course over these next few weeks and view your BBC experience not only as a health and fitness makeover, but as a turning point that reconnects you with your deepest self and empowers you to continue making positive changes in all areas of your life.

There's something about being on an expansive, sun-drenched beach in Mexico that enables us to see our lives more clearly. Far removed from the trappings of twenty-first-century living, our guests are able to enjoy the kind of introspection and solace that their busy schedules back home rarely afford. In putting the Bikini Bootcamp program into a book, our greatest challenge was how to capture that tranquility and peace of mind that our campers experience at Amansala and translate it into something you can find wherever you are. When the noise and chaos of everyday life subside, our guests are able to listen to their bodies and truly relish the changes that are taking place. That sense of inner calm and refreshed perspective, not to mention joy at how their bodies are transforming before their eyes, is what spurs them to stick with the program even when it's tough, and to keep up with the changes they've made when they say good-bye.

With that in mind, we've put together several daily exercises to help you find the same inner quietude, connect with how your body is feeling, and encourage yourself to stay on the right track. For each day, in addition to the prescribed workouts and recipes, you'll find a Daily Inspiration, a journal-writing exercise, and a meditation. Do you *need* to do these exercises to lose weight and get fit? No, but they will greatly enhance the journey you're about to take. In addition to calming and centering you, they will help you remain focused on your goals and give you results that go far beyond a terrific shape.

Daily Inspirations

Your daily inspiration is a word, concept, or idea designed to motivate you throughout your day. It may be something you need to cultivate for yourself, like patience or flexibility, or something you want to extend to others, like gratitude. Every day at Bikini Bootcamp, we post a daily inspiration on our chalkboard to serve as food for thought. Usually it goes hand in hand with your journal-writing exercise, so use them together to explore different thoughts, feelings, questions, dreams, and what you want your life to look like when these two weeks are up.

Journal Writing

Your Bikini Bootcamp journal is not a food diary or exercise log. It is reflective writing and, hopefully, a wonderful tool for keeping an eye on your goals. In Mexico, our guests assemble on the beach first thing in the morning to write in their journals *in silence* for at least fifteen minutes. These journals are private—not for sharing, even with friends and loved ones. Your writing can take any form—poetry, stories, lists, traditional diary entries, or anything else that comes to you and helps you clear your mind and focus on the day that lies ahead. It's important for you to trust the process and enjoy the freedom to express yourself fully. There are no rules, so don't be concerned with the content or grammar. Just see whatever you produce as a stream of consciousness. Journals are great listeners: Between their covers you can set loose your fears, share secrets, and confess your innermost desires without worrying about what anyone thinks.

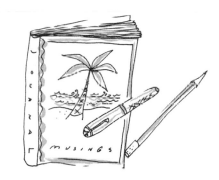

The act of writing is also one of the best ways to clear your mind of unnecessary clutter from the past. Once you get started, you will find that releasing any old thoughts, issues, or emotions onto the paper frees you to let them go. When you're embarking on a lifestyle change, it is incredibly useful to identify any lingering beliefs—about you, about your body, about what you are capable of—that have been keeping you stuck in a fitness and dieting rut. Now is the time to get them out of your head and onto the page. Believe it or not, once you purge excess baggage from your mind, it becomes easier to purge excess weight from your body, too. Clear minds create clear bodies!

As journal writing becomes your daily ritual, you will come to cherish this activity as a sacred intermission from your busy life and a wonderful opportunity to focus on what's really important. Many of the same guests who were reluctant to even try the Bikini Bootcamp journal (some more vocal in their protests than others!) were amazed after they returned home to find that they were still writing every day. By giving themselves a few "rules"—a specific time of day to journal, a quiet spot, and a specific time limit—and by knowing their writing was entirely private, they were able to tap into deeper levels of creativity and clarity. As one camper, Allison, put it, "Bikini Bootcamp journal writing really helped me slow down and recognize automatic but unconscious habits—like reaching for a cookie every time I sat in front of the TV—that were keeping me from losing weight as well as from reaching my true potential in other aspects of my life." One of our other campers, Beth, wrote to us a few months after she did the program, "BBC journal writing helped me to take better care of myself as I became more in tune with my real feelings and my desire to lose weight and get in shape."

When our guests arrive at Bikini Bootcamp, we ask them to do an introductory journal exercise to set their intentions for the week. We recommend that you do the same, so grab a pen and a sheet of paper, and ask yourself two important questions, the same questions that all our BBC attendees gather around in a circle to answer on the night of their arrival:

• Why am I undertaking the Bikini Bootcamp program?
• What exactly do I want to achieve?

As you write down your answers, do so with blunt honesty. Remember, no one is looking over your shoulder, and no one but you will ever see your responses. Even if parts of your answers seem pointless or vague, write down everything that comes to mind until you have come to the ones that resound within you as true.

Believe it or not, asking and then answering these simple questions is the beginning of a life-changing process, because writing down your goals and intentions is the first step in making them a reality. Keep these intentions close at hand and revisit them every day, revising and updating them as necessary. You can have short-term intentions that are as basic as committing to doing all of the activities for that day's program: "Today, I will do my one-hour walk, my yoga practice, circuit training, and core strengthening. I will eat only what is on the day's menu." Or, you can set goals for what you want to achieve by the end of the two weeks: "I want to lose five pounds, I want to see my abs, and I want to feel great when I see myself in the mirror." Even "I want to be on a new path to looking and feeling healthier" is an excellent intention to inspire you in the weeks ahead. But you should try to set some long-term goals as well—for one, five, or even ten or more years from now—because they will provide additional clarity and purpose to your life and motivate you to stay fit, slim, and healthy long after your new bikini has gone out of style.

Though it's best to start off each day with several minutes of Bikini Bootcamp journal writing, even before you shower and dress, journaling can be done on the subway on your way to work, during your coffee break, waiting in line at the bank, or anyplace and anytime a window opens in your schedule for quiet private time in which you can let your thoughts flow onto the paper. Remember: This is not a food or exercise journal, although your thoughts, concerns, and goals about eating and exercising are certainly good journaling topics. But even if you never write a single word about exercise or food, after a relatively brief time of regular Bikini Bootcamp journal writing, you will discover that you are more connected to your real self, your real needs, and your body. We are constantly amazed by the number of guests who leave Bikini Bootcamp not only thinner and more toned, but also happier—because they've finally taken the time to hear their own thoughts, get clarity on what they want for their futures, and let go of whatever limitations they once imposed on themselves.

Places to Squeeze in BBC Journaling Time

On the bus, train, or subway to and from work
Waiting for an appointment
Waiting for a late friend
During a morning or afternoon break
Just before bed
Anytime, anyplace at all!

Meditation

If you're searching for a cure for the everyday stress and anxiety that can leave you feeling tired and frazzled, and threaten to derail your Bikini

Bootcamp experience ("I can't possibly walk for an hour today—I have no time!"), look no further than this wonderfully calming practice and powerful tool. Meditation isn't about renouncing the world or sitting in an uncomfortable position for hours while you try to "empty your mind." It's simply a great way to slow down, breathe, let all your cares and worries fall away, be in the present moment, and refocus so you can get the results that you want.

Like journaling, meditation clears your mind and increases self-awareness. And just like yoga, meditation is a practice, which means that over time you become better at it. So even if you're a meditation skeptic, or the kind of girl who *never* sits still, even for a minute, we urge you to give it a try.

The quickie beginners' meditations that are slotted into each of the fourteen days in Part II can be practiced in just ten minutes or even less so that you stay on your BBC track. Even in this brief amount of time, they allow you to observe the thoughts that occupy your mental space, recognize if those thoughts are positive or negative, and release them. As you practice meditation consistently, you will find it easier and easier to observe yourself from a clearer and more objective perspective. Our Bikini Bootcampers love the soothing and meditative effects of focusing on the rhythm of the waves crashing on the shore, but you can get the same relaxing benefits by paying attention to the sounds of your own inhalations and exhalations, even while you're sitting in traffic.

One of the greatest benefits of regular meditation is that as you become more aware, you no longer have to engage in negative behaviors—like overeating or choosing to "veg out" on the couch rather than going outdoors and exercising—to avoid uncomfortable thoughts and feelings. Instead, you recognize the feelings when they surface and simply release them and let them go.

During our group meditation at Bikini Bootcamp, we give our campers an example to illustrate the importance of living in the present moment. Monkeys who swing through the jungle from tree to tree hold on to a branch behind them with one hand until they are ready to move forward. But in order to move from one branch to another they must let go of the branch behind them fully and surrender to that moment of free space before they can grab hold of the next one out in front of them. The same is true of all of us. In order to move forward, you have to let go of the past—all the excuses and rationalizations and anything else that's keeping you stuck—so you can move freely toward the life you want, one in which you are healthy, fit, and comfortable with yourself, your body, and your circumstances. By practicing the meditations in Part II, you will learn to embrace the present so you truly feel as though you are starting a new chapter of your life.

This subtle but all-important action of being present and aware can make everything you do on the BBC program—from circuit training to core strengthening to yoga—more effective and give you even greater results. So bring a little meditation mindfulness to your workouts! You'll also become more involved in the activity so that you truly enjoy it rather than just go through the motions. We hope that over these next two weeks you will come to do *all* the elements of the Bikini Bootcamp program with your whole heart and mind. In this way you're guaranteed not only to see your body transform, but to actually have fun in the process.

Tips for Meditation

We recommend that you try each of the ten-minute meditations in Part II at least once. You are free to rotate among them, choosing a different one for each day. Or, if you prefer, stick to your favorite meditation practice throughout the next two weeks. Here are some other tips to guide you.

- Find a comfortable meditation place. Experiment with different spots to discover which is best for you.
- Turn off the TV and the telephone ringer.
- Breathe in and out, paying attention to the feeling of the air as it enters and exits. Make sure you are breathing slowly and deeply.
- As thoughts arise, simply acknowledge them and let them go. Imagine that your thoughts are floating down a river, and you are sitting on the bank, observing, not reaching out to grab any of them, but just letting them float on by.

Ten Minutes of Daily Meditation Gives You . . .

Clarity of mind to make the right food and exercise choices.

Sense of balance and centeredness to keep you on the Bikini Bootcamp track.

Feelings of calm and overall well-being.

Lower blood pressure for greater exercise capacity.

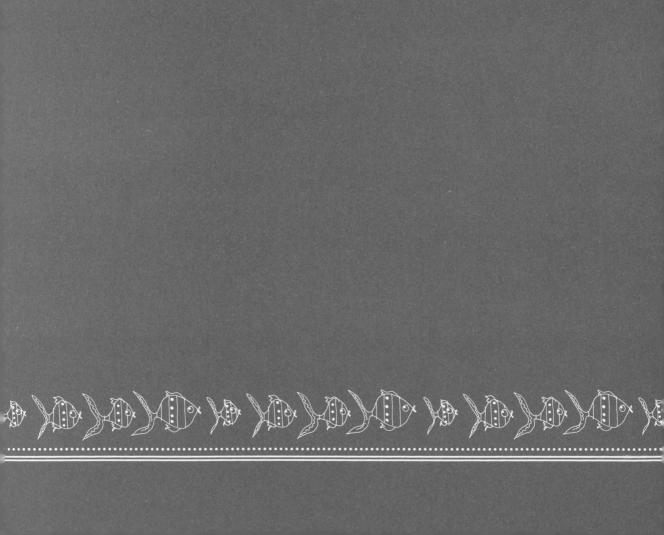

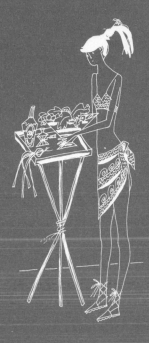

PART II

The Program

The beginning is always today.

—*Mary Wollstonecraft Shelley*

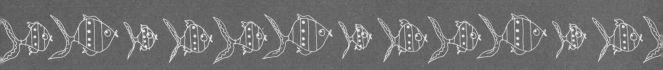

$\mathcal{N}\text{ow}$ that you've read Part I and learned how the Bikini Bootcamp components work together to give you a head-to-toe, body-sculpting makeover, you are ready to put everything into action at last.

Bikini Bootcamp is about challenging yourself and pushing old, worn-out boundaries. Yes, you'll be asked to step out of your comfort zone—whether it's about making new food choices or moving your body—but don't be intimidated! You picked up this book for a reason, and starting today, it's time to make your ultimate beach body a reality . . . inside and out.

For many of you, this may well be more exercise than you've ever done in a day, and you will be eating in a way you may never have experienced. So let's be honest—it's not going to be easy! There will probably be times when you're tempted to throw in the towel and skip your circuit training, or reach for a sugary snack. But if you approach this program with a commitment to yourself and to sticking with it for just these next two weeks, before you know it you'll be seeing results, and that will spur you to stay the course. Soon you'll be reaching for those skinny jeans that have been hanging in the back of your closet for far too long, and feeling great when you step into that bikini to hit the pool. Our hope is that you'll start to think of exercise as a reward before or after a long day at the office, and wholesome, delicious food as a gift you give yourself because you know that you—and your body—are worth it.

Your only job from here on is to follow the Bikini Bootcamp program we've laid out for you each day. Each element of the program, from your daily workouts to the meal plans, is outlined in an easy-to-follow manner. We've also included a "spa treat" suggestion for each day, plus plenty of helpful tips, information, and inspiration scattered throughout for extra motivation whenever you need it.

Keep in mind as you go that what you put into the program is what you will get out of it. Know your limits and rest when you need to, but don't be afraid to challenge yourself. Simply stick to each day's plan and refer to Parts I and III whenever you need a reminder of the hows and whys behind any part of the workouts, recipes, or other elements. So are you ready for your bikini body? Then let's get started!

Getting Started

Before you make your fresh start on Day 1, be sure you have the following equipment:

- Yoga mat (or exercise mat, or towel)
- Three- to five-pound hand weights (or soup cans, water bottles, or whatever else you have available)
- Jump rope (optional)
- Towel
- Comfortable workout clothes
- Cross trainers or aerobic shoes
- Journal and pen

Find a Bootcamp Buddy

Sticking with a new weight loss and exercise regimen is markedly easier—not to mention more fun—if you have at least one partner in crime. At Bikini Bootcamp there's strength in numbers: Our guests eat together, work out together, and gather in the evenings to gab and laugh about their sore muscles and celebrate each other's successes. If you can, find a friend and do BBC together, so you can share your triumphs, no matter how small they may be, like the fact that you finally did Circuit A in the optimum thirty-eight minutes, or turned down a brownie during your afternoon coffee break. Make sure you keep each other motivated even after you graduate BBC. After all, this is just the beginning! If you can't find a friend to share your journey, make your journal your first success partner and use it to chronicle all the terrific strides you make.

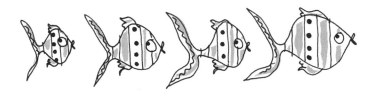

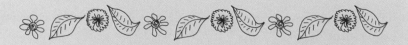

A Sensory Experience

In Mexico, the tantalizing scent of ocean air and tropical flowers keeps us feeling refreshed and energized. But even if you're a city dweller, you can re-create the feel of Bikini Bootcamp by using scented candles and essential oils. You'll experience the benefits immediately because the properties of essential oils penetrate beyond the blood-brain barrier. Medical studies have even found that depressed people who sniffed citrus odors needed less antidepressants to feel better! Try these known mood-lifters for extra energy and a fragrant treat while you're on the BBC regimen:

Orange

Lemon

Tangerine

Clary sage

Geranium

Peppermint

Rose

Ylang-ylang

Clove

Vanilla

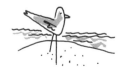

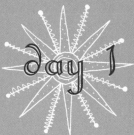

day 1

Each decision we make, each action we take, is born out of intention.
—*Sharon Salzberg*

Journal Writing
Morning Meditation: Ten-Minute Breath
Yoga: 15 minutes of Sun Salutations
Walking: 30 minutes to an hour at a brisk pace
Circuit Training: Circuit A
Core Strengthening: Series A

Welcome to your very first day of Bikini Bootcamp! Today marks the start of your unique total-body transformation, inside and out. If you've been fretting about the numbers on the scale, don't worry—you're about to take action. And you'll be ready to hit the beach in just two weeks!

As you begin the program, keep in mind that the many different components may seem overwhelming at first. You're going to be using new muscles, thinking in new ways, and trying new recipes, maybe with ingredients you've never used before. Adjusting to the increased level of activity may be a challenge as well. You might find yourself wondering if you'll *ever* manage to make it through the complete circuit training workout. But trust us when we tell you to stay the course. It *will* get easier, and before you know it, the pounds will start disappearing. There's

nothing like positive reinforcement to keep you moving and eating right!

TODAY'S INSPIRATION IS INTENTION

Starting today, you want to recognize the intense power of your thoughts to effect real changes in your life. Take some time to set your intentions as described in Chapter 6. Visualize what you are seeking—a slimmer, more toned figure; more energy; and more confidence in who you are—and believe that it is possible.

JOURNAL WRITING

As soon as you wake up, open your new journal and write for at least 15 minutes. Remember: Your journal is a great listener. Between its covers you can set loose your fears, share your secrets, and claim your dreams in unedited stream-of-consciousness writing that no one but you will ever read. If possible, journal before you do anything else so you can clear your mind of all the clutter, fears, and doubts that may prevent you from seizing the day and fully immersing yourself in the Bikini Bootcamp program. Be sure to include your intentions and goals for the next two weeks as well as any long-term goals. But remember that your life is happening NOW; it does not start once your goals are met, so live each day to the fullest, and keep in mind that today's intentions are not set in stone.

MORNING MEDITATION:
Ten-Minute Breath

This powerfully calming and centering beginner's meditation takes only 10 minutes to decompress you from even the most frazzled moments, and you can practice it for a longer period if you choose. Meditation is a great way to start your day. Or it can mark the end of a busy day and the beginning of a relaxing evening and a good night's rest. Remember that you can meditate anytime, especially when stress threatens to sabotage your commitment to BBC.

1.   Find a comfortable seat. Traditionally, we sit in a crossed-legged position for meditation, but if your knees are bothering you or if you suffer from any injuries that make this position uncomfortable, try lying on your back or sitting in a chair instead. The idea is to find a position that you will be comfortable in for a while. If you are sitting in a crossed-legged position, place your hands on your knees,

palms facing down, to symbolize that all you need is within you already. If you are lying down, place your right hand on your heart and your left hand on your belly.

2.   Allow your tongue to rest on the roof of your mouth and begin to establish your breathing by becoming aware of your breath. For many of us, becoming aware of our breath is a very new concept. Yes, we breathe in and out all the time, but we do it unconsciously, with little awareness.

3.   Now inhale and exhale through your nose. Do not hold your breath. Instead allow your mind to follow your pattern of inhalations and exhalations. Imagine energy flooding your body with each inhalation, and then let go of any impurities or negative thoughts with each exhalation, creating space for fresh oxygen to come in. As thoughts come into your mind, acknowledge them and then let them go. Imagine these thoughts floating by you on a passing cloud as your mind clears. Recognize that all that matters is the present moment symbolized by each breath. Continue in this way for 10 minutes.

YOGA: 15 Minutes of
Sun Salutations

For the optimum Bikini Bootcamp experience, you should follow your journaling and meditation with 15 minutes or more of Sun Salutations, topped off with the *pranayama* of your choice—Alternate

The best way to cultivate your daily walking habit is to keep your walking clothes and shoes by the front door at home or in a desk drawer at your office, so you can change into them as soon as you get home or whenever you break during the day for lunch. For those days when you don't feel like walking, tell yourself you will just take a few steps or make your way down to the end of your street and back. Once you get started, you'll soon find yourself craving to do your full session.

Nostril Breathing if you feel frazzled, or the Fire Breath if you need an energy boost. If your schedule makes this impossible, don't worry, but be sure to find time for your 15 minutes—or more of yoga, plus a breathing exercise, at some point during each day.

BEGINNERS: Work at a slower pace and do not worry about the number of Sun Salutations you complete. Take your time to become familiar with the breathing pattern, the *asanas* (postures), and your body's response.

INTERMEDIATE AND ADVANCED: Start slowly and gradually increase the pace and the number of times you repeat the sequence, but only to a point where you can maintain the connection to your breath and your body's movements.

WALKING: 30 Minutes to 1 Hour

In an ideal world, you would take your walk in the morning, immediately after journaling, meditation, and yoga. But we know this is not possible for many of you, so anytime during the day or evening is fine. You can also schedule your walking time in brief spurts of no less than 10 minutes throughout the day to fit into your daily routine, as long as you move at a good pace.

The first time you set out for your walk is always the hardest, but it gets easier from there. Whenever possible, walk outdoors in fresh air so you can connect to your environment and the day as well as make use of the challenges offered by outdoor terrain. If there's a park nearby, head straight for it, but a few times

Remember, when doing yoga, link your breath to your movements so it's fluid and rhythmic. Never, ever hold your breath.

around your block is also fine. An added benefit of the daily outdoor walk is the community you will discover among other walkers, joggers, and runners.

BEGINNERS: If you are currently out of the walking habit, start out walking for 30 minutes minimum, and then build up incrementally as directed in the days that follow.

ADVANCED: Start out by walking for the full hour. Rev up the calorie burn with a weighted vest (remember, holding weights or strapping them to your ankles can increase the risk of injury).

CIRCUIT TRAINING: Circuit A

We're going to start off with Circuit Training regimen A (found on page 24). Remember: Don't count reps when you're doing a circuit. Do watch the clock. Your goal for the next 14 days is to work your way up to completing 2 rounds of the circuit within 38 minutes. Keep moving as quickly as possible while maintaining proper form, allowing 15 seconds of setup between each exercise.

CORE STRENGTHENING: Series A

Though you won't be doing a core strength series every day, we're going to jump-start your sexy abs makeover on Day One. For your core strength exercises, you only need your mat. Make sure you read through the workout (found on page 59) several times so you'll have a clear sense of how to do the exercises.

TODAY'S MEAL PLAN

MORNING BURST: The first thing to pass through your mouth every day should be 1 cup of hot water with a squeeze of fresh lemon

BREAKFAST: Blueberry Smoothie (page 209)

LUNCH: Amansala Salad with Grilled Fish & Ginger-Sesame Dressing (page 215)

SNACK: Jicama sticks with a squeeze of a slice of lime & a pinch of salt

DINNER: Tortilla-less Tortilla Soup (page 235)

Chicken Fajitas with Black Beans, Guacamole & Salsa Mexicana (page 241)

DESSERT: Fruit Kebabs (page 253)

Bikini Tip
Remember to breathe! In yoga, we inhale and exhale through the nose, practicing *ujjayi* breathing. But in circuit training and core strengthening, just breathe normally and naturally—inhaling through your nose and exhaling through your mouth.

Eat one meal today in total silence (without a book to read or the TV on). Take time to notice the details of your meal. How does the food smell? How does it feel in your mouth? How does it taste? How many times do you chew? How is your stomach reacting to what is going on? If you're keeping a temporary food diary, you can note these observations in your journal.

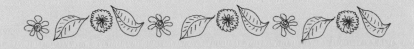

Cooling Cucumber & Honey Scalp Treatment

What's a bikini body without great hair? This soothing, all-natural scalp treatment nourishes your hair for a fuller, shinier feel. The only living part of your hair—the bulb—is rooted in the scalp, so it follows that for your hair to look good, your scalp must be in optimum condition. This treatment has all the right ingredients to cool, soothe, and moisturize the skin beneath your mane. It feels luscious and can be made in your own kitchen—much cheaper than a trip to the salon.

  1/4 cucumber, peeled

  1 kiwi (peeled)

  1/2 cup of plain yogurt

  1 large serving of honey/tablespoon size

Puree the cucumber and kiwi, and then mix with yogurt and honey. Apply the mixture carefully to dry hair, smoothing it on so that every hair and every inch of your scalp are thoroughly coated. Leave for 10 minutes, then shampoo.

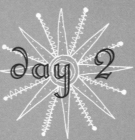

day 2

Success is focusing the full power of all you are on what
you have a burning desire to achieve.

—*Wilferd A. Peterson*

Journal Writing
Morning Meditation: De-Stress
Yoga: 15 minutes of Sun Salutations
Walking: 30 minutes to 1 hour at a brisk pace
Circuit Training: Circuit B

Welcome to Day 2! You may be feeling sore and a bit tired from yesterday's activities, but you should also be reveling in your new acquaintance with muscles you may have never even known you had! You've got one day of healthy, gourmet dining under your shrinking belt, so keep it up! Be proud of yourself and stay excited about this new journey. You are one day closer to your goal.

TODAY'S INSPIRATION IS MINDFULNESS

Mindfulness means that you are fully aware and present in each moment, so every activity—from eating to driving to talking on the phone with a friend—becomes an opportunity to be fully awake and alive. You're paying attention to the world around you, noticing how it makes you feel. As you flow through your day,

remind yourself to be mindful of each activity you undertake.

JOURNAL WRITING

Write in your journal for 15 minutes. Remember: If you're too busy in the morning, evenings are also a good time to journal because you can get any frustrations, worries, or other concerns that pile up during your day out of your head and onto paper, thus clearing the way for a restful, restorative night's sleep. Do not overthink your journal entries—just write!

MORNING MEDITATION: De-Stress

Tension may begin in the mind, but it often lodges in your body, adding to your physical stress load even when you are feeling mentally at ease. This meditation allows you to scan your body and pinpoint exactly where you are holding tension, so you have the option to let it go.

1. Sit down somewhere comfortable and close your eyes. Take a few deep inhalations through your nose and exhale through your mouth.
2. Continuing to breathe deeply, focus on the top of your head and your forehead, sensing any tension and giving it permission to let go.
3. Move progressively down through the rest of your body, from your neck to your shoulders on down, sensing any tension in each group of muscles and letting it go.
4. After you finish, take a quick inventory of any muscles still holding tension and let it go.

YOGA: 15 Minutes of Sun Salutations

BEGINNERS: Remember to work at a slower pace and don't be concerned with the number of Sun Salutation sequences you complete. Instead, continue to become familiar with *ujjayi* breathing, the *asanas* (postures), and your body's response.

INTERMEDIATE AND ADVANCED: Continue increasing the pace and number of repetitions, but only to a point where you still maintain a connection to your breath and body. Remember: Yoga is not a competitive sport! If you want some variety, mix your flow up by incorporating some of the extra postures on pages 103–106 at the end of your flow sequence.

Ease your way back to "real life" by ending with the *pranayama* of your choice.

WALKING: 30 Minutes to 1 Hour

Make sure you find time for your daily walk. Even if you're not concerned with losing weight, walking does build muscle and provide terrific cardiovascular benefits, so be sure you walk for at least 30 minutes.

CIRCUIT TRAINING: Circuit B

Repeat each exercise in Circuit B (found on page 33) for the allotted time, aiming for perfect form. Remember, do not count reps! Also remember that whenever you are doing any kind of exercise, you should never lock your knees and elbows. Keep them slightly soft but controlled, to prevent joint injury.

TODAY'S MEAL PLAN

MORNING BURST: Hot water with lemon
BREAKFAST: Banana Swirl (page 208)
LUNCH: Chopped Vegetable & Chickpea Salad with Citrus Dressing (page 218)
SNACK: 10 whole almonds with one tbsp. raisins
DINNER: Mushroom Spinach Soup (page 232)

Bikini Tip: Walk on Grass
Head for your backyard or the nearest park and stroll through the dewy morning grass to feel especially energized and grounded.

Grilled Ginger Shrimp with Zucchini (page 246)

DESSERT: Baked Apple with Brown Sugar & Cinnamon (page 251)

Avocado Madness

At Bikini Bootcamp, we love avocados, and not just for eating! This versatile fruit is packed with protein and natural oils and rich in Vitamins A, B, and E, so it's as good for your inside as your outside. In some countries, women apply mashed avocado straight to their faces and hair for protection and moisturizing. And in fact, avocado oil is found in many high-end beauty products, including some of those made by Bobbi Brown. No matter what condition your hair or skin is in, these deluxe avocado treatments will bring you back to soft, smooth balance. Here are our own back-to-basic twists:

FOR YOUR HAIR Mash 1 overripe avocado until it looks ready for guacamole. Mix in 1 egg yolk and 2 tablespoons of olive oil. Massage into damp hair and tuck under a shower cap. Leave on for 20 minutes, and then rinse, shampoo, and condition.

FOR DRY SKIN Apply raw avocado that's been mashed with a fork immediately to the affected area. Leave on for 15 minutes, and then rinse with warm water.

FOR OILY SKIN Add 1 egg white to the mashed flesh of avocado and apply to your face. Leave on for 15 minutes, and then rinse with warm water.

FOR COMBINATION SKIN Add 1 lightly beaten egg yolk to a mashed half avocado and apply to your face. Leave on for 15 minutes, and then rinse with warm water.

FOR MATURE SKIN Add 1 tablespoon of honey to one mashed avocado and apply to your face. Leave on for 15 minutes, and then rinse with warm water.

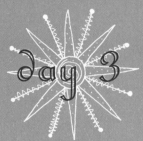

day 3

Far away in the sunshine are my highest aspirations. I may not reach them, but I can look up and see their beauty, believe in them, and try to follow where they lead.

—*Louisa May Alcott*

Journal Writing
Morning Meditation: Tonglin
Yoga: 15 Minutes of Sun Salutations
Walking: 30 minutes to 1 hour at a brisk pace
Circuit Training: Circuit C
Core Strengthening: Series B

Only twelve more days to go before you hit the beach in your bikini! You've accomplished two days of healthy eating and moving your body, and you may have felt tired at the end of each day, but we're betting that it's a "good" tired, not a "stressed-out" one. You're well on your way to a new life in which you take great care of yourself and look and feel your best.

TODAY'S INSPIRATION IS COMPASSION

Today, remember to hold compassion not only for others, but also for *you!* We are often our own worst critics, and an insistence on meeting an impossible ideal of perfection can sabotage your efforts to complete BBC successfully. Allow yourself room to fail and to fall as you work to overcome life's challenges. Maybe you're struggling with the circuit training—that's okay! Know that it—like all aspects of the program—will get easier with time. You also want to be sure to extend the same compassion to others. We often do not know the circumstances that make people who they are or explain why they act a certain way. Often their behavior has nothing to do with us, but with what happened fifteen minutes, two days, or even ten years ago. Keep this in mind, because the less negative energy you take on and carry around, the better!

JOURNAL WRITING

Keep your Daily Inspiration of Compassion in mind as you let your thoughts flow onto the paper today. If you want guidance in this exercise, you can ask yourself the following questions:

- Am I holding compassion for myself, or do I have the habit of judging myself negatively?
- Do I forgive myself for my failures and then move on, or do I stay stuck in self-condemnation?
- Do I hold compassion for others, or do I judge them harshly and react defensively when I believe I've been treated wrongly?
- What can I do, starting today, to be a more compassionate person?

MORNING MEDITATION: Tonglin

The goal of this simple meditation is to transform any self-defeating thoughts into positive energy.

1. Come to a comfortable seated position. Think of someone or something that needs your positive thoughts. This can be anything or anyone, from the poor in Africa to a friend suffering from a broken heart. It can even include yourself and your need for encouragement during BBC.
2. Inhale through your nose, imagining that you are drawing in all the negativity, pain, and suffering that surround this person or situation.
3. As you exhale again through your nose, imagine that you are transforming all that negativity into peace, love, compassion, hope, positive thoughts, and energy for this person or situation.
4. Follow this breathing pattern for at least five breaths, holding in your mind the person/situation.

YOGA: 15 Minutes of Sun Salutations

If some of the poses still feel new and strange, that's normal, so be patient—as your muscles get stronger and more flexible, the flow will come more easily. Yoga is a personal journey; so remember, never compare your practice to anyone else's.

BEGINNERS: Continue working at a slower pace and don't be concerned with the number of Sun Salutation sequences you complete. Instead, continue to become familiar with *ujjayi* breathing, the *asanas* (postures), and your body's response.

INTERMEDIATE AND ADVANCED: Continue increasing the pace and number of repetitions, but only to a point where you still maintain a connection to your breath and body. If you want some variety, mix up your flow by incorporating some of the extra postures on pages 103–106 to the end of your flow sequence.

Bikini Tip

Eat at the table, not standing up or while engaged in other activities. Our tendency to gobble food on the go, in front of the television, or at our desks makes it easy to overeat because we're distracted from our bodies' signals of hunger and fullness. Sitting at the table so you can relish your food actually helps you eat less.

Ease your way back to "real life" by ending with the *pranayama* of your choice.

WALKING: 30 MINUTES TO 1 HOUR

To make sure you're getting the most out of your walk, review the instructions and illustrations for proper posture given in Chapter 4. There's a direct correlation between your form and the results you'll see. Again, when you are doing any kind of exercise, never lock your knees or elbows. Always keep them slightly soft, but controlled, in order to prevent joint injury.

CIRCUIT TRAINING: Circuit C

Remember to work at a steady pace, using the clock to tell you when to stop one exercise and go on to the next one. Use your favorite music to keep you energized and moving.

CORE STRENGTHENING: Series B

Sense how your waist is already whittling down with these torso-targeting moves and know that you will be in bikini-ready shape in no time!

TODAY'S MEAL PLAN

MORNING BURST: Hot water with lemon
BREAKFAST: Mango Yogurt Parfait (page 212)
LUNCH: White Bean & Tuna Salad in Orange-Cilantro Dressing (page 223)
SNACK: Carrot sticks with hummus (page 266)
DINNER: White Bean & Roasted Tomato Soup (page 236)
Curried Spinach Salad with Grilled Chicken, Papaya & Pumpkin Seeds (page 220)
DESSERT: Fresh pineapple

Bath with Essential Oils

There's no better way to unwind after a long day full of responsibilities and exercise than with a hot bath. For best results, take your bath an hour before bedtime and soak for no longer than 30 minutes. Add a few drops of your preferred essential oil, such as lavender or chamomile, to help you relax and unwind. If you don't have either of these oils on hand, add a few chamomile tea bags to the hot water instead. Enhance your at-home spa experience by rolling a bath towel and placing it under your neck and then scattering lit candles around your bathtub. Relax and enjoy!

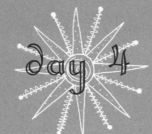

day 4

Happiness is a process, not a destination.
—*Anonymous*

Journal Writing
Morning Meditation: Mindful Walking
Yoga: 15 minutes of Sun Salutations
Walking: 30 minutes to 1 hour at a brisk pace
Circuit Training: Circuit A

By now you should be getting the hang of things and feeling more energized and confident. You may already have noticed your belly flattening and your legs feeling tighter. Yes, you're probably sore, but this is "sweet pain," the kind that accompanies great changes. As you continue through this day and the rest of Bikini Bootcamp, you'll feel stronger and stronger and see your body transforming into the ideal shape you've always dreamed of.

TODAY'S INSPIRATION IS GRATITUDE
Count your blessings! There are so many gifts to be thankful for that we often overlook them in the business of our daily lives, especially when we are feeling stressed out and sorry for ourselves.

Which can only lead to trouble . . . and the refrigerator. Bikini Bootcamp is all about empowerment. You're taking charge of your life by eating and exercising, and yes, even thinking positively can help you fulfill these goals. As you move through your day, take a moment here and there to remember why you are grateful. Above all, remember to be grateful for your body, and that you are able to move and exercise and enjoy this experience of becoming fit and healthy.

JOURNAL WRITING
Take this opportunity to start a gratitude section of your journal by writing down at least five things for which you are thankful, even if it's as simple as, "I can breathe." Gratitude lifts you from any negativity and sets you back on course.

From now on, every time you eat, whether it's a quick snack or a full-course dinner, ask the universe to infuse your food with nourishment and energy and express your gratitude for the food. You'll enjoy your meals more by being fully in the present and probably wind up eating less.

MORNING MEDITATION:
Mindful Walking

Practice the following meditation during your walk today. Walk in silence—no music, no friend, no cell phone—and allow your walk to become a chance to quiet the constant commentary that runs through your mind. Be mindful of your breath as well as the sounds and sights around you. If you typically walk indoors on a treadmill, take your walk outside, if weather permits, and enjoy all of nature's little gifts.

YOGA: 15 Minutes of Sun Salutations

BEGINNERS: Do your 15 minutes or more of Sun Salutations, and add a lunge sequence from the next level, if you feel ready.

INTERMEDIATE AND ADVANCED: Keep your flow even and steady and work up to a quicker pace. Try some of the extra *asanas* listed in Chapter 3.

At the end, take a few minutes to practice any of the *pranayamas* listed in Chapter 3.

WALKING: 30 Minutes to 1 Hour

Remember to do today's Mindful Walking Meditation and leave that iPod or cell phone at home!

CIRCUIT TRAINING: CIRCUIT A

Remember to keep your eye on the clock and your pace steady.

TODAY'S MEAL PLAN

MORNING BURST: Hot water with lemon
BREAKFAST: Huevos Mexicana (page 210)
LUNCH: Chicken Taco Salad (page 217)
SNACK: 1 cup low-fat plain or vanilla yogurt with 1 tbsp. raisins
DINNER: Carrot Ginger Soup (page 228) Fish Kebabs with Zucchini, Mushrooms & Cherry Tomatoes (page 243)
DESSERT: Watermelon Frappé (page 256)

Green Tea Spritz

Brew a cup or two of green tea and, when it cools, pour it into a mini spray bottle, then store it in the fridge. Enjoy a few spritzes of cool tea on your flushed and overheated skin after your workout. The tea is rich in anti-inflammatory agents and it soothes your skin, leaving you looking rejuvenated and refreshed rather than hot and winded.

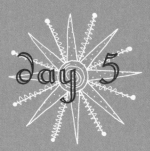

day 5

Self-confidence is the first requisite to great undertakings.

—*Samuel Johnson*

Journal Writing
Morning Meditation: Full Body Meditation
Yoga: 15 minutes of Sun Salutations
Walking: 45 minutes to 1 hour
Circuit Training: Circuit B
Core Strengthening: Series A

Okay, okay, you're a bit tired and your muscles ache. Just take a moment to switch your focus to something better—the beach and you looking fabulous in your bikini. So, welcome to Day 5! By now you're practically a BBC pro, and your work colleagues, friends, and family may have noticed something's different. They may not know exactly what the change is, but they like it. And you've got a mirror: Can't you see that your skin's glowing, and your pants may even be a bit looser? Forward in every direction!

TODAY'S INSPIRATION IS DISCOVERY

Bikini Bootcamp is all about discovering this amazing gift that you have been given—your body. The way it moves, its abilities . . . even its limitations. BBC is also about RE-discovering parts of yourself you may have neglected or forgotten, including your spirit and passion—everything that makes your heart sing. Today, let your Bikini Bootcamp progress be the impetus for discovering changes you may want to make in other areas of your life.

JOURNAL WRITING

For today's journal, jot down some thoughts about discoveries you have made over the past few days—from your tight hamstrings to your newly toned abs to your realization that you might actually like fish or vegetables! Write about what these discoveries have inspired, and other life changes you may want to make.

MORNING MEDITATION:
Full Body Meditation

Start your day *before* you get out of bed with this quick and easy relaxer:

1. Lie on your back with your eyes closed, and your arms by your sides, your palms facing up. Begin by breathing comfortably, but with awareness.

2. Once you have established a regular pattern of inhalations and exhalations, begin to mentally explore your body, keeping your eyes closed. Begin by feeling your feet. Imagine what they look like when viewed from above. Allow them to feel heavy, secure on the earth beneath you.

3. Follow this pattern as you move, part by part, up your entire body, ending at the crown of your head.

YOGA: 15 Minutes
of Sun Salutations

BEGINNERS: By now, the repetitive movements of the Sun Salutations and *ujjayi* breath (traditional yogic breath inhaling in and out of the nose) will be a bit more familiar, so you can begin to experiment with the pace. Pick up the speed of your routine a bit, but not so much that you lose the proper form. Continue exploring the breath, the *asanas* (postures), and your body. Try adding one of the extra *asanas* from pages 103–106 to the end of your flow sequence just for fun!

INTERMEDIATE AND ADVANCED: You can increase the pace as well, but only to a point where you can still maintain a connection to your body and your breath. Continue to mix up the flow by incorporating some of the postures from the next level or the extra *asanas* on pages 103–106

Bikini Tip

To up the cardio factor of your walks, try to choose *safe* routes with varied terrain, especially hills, which increase the benefit to your heart and lungs, give your butt an extra workout, and keep your mind alert. Uphill walking is great exercise. Not only do you increase the caloric burn, but it's also easy on your knees and tightens your butt, thighs, and lower legs. When walking uphill, try to keep the intensity level equal to the rest of your walk. Walk as flat-footed as you can, but don't lock your knees as you step; this way your weight and effort will be in your thighs instead of your calves. If your route has no hills, get creative. Trails may provide a softer surface and a beautiful environment, but you can also add a little challenge to your walk by climbing up and down stairs or parking lot ramps, or walking across arching bridges. When coming down, take smaller, controlled steps to minimize the risk of injury. If you use a treadmill, do high-intensity speed intervals and hill climbing in rapid succession, letting the treadmill's absorbable surface reduce the impact. Every 3 minutes add 1-minute incline intervals by raising the incline to a level that allows you to work harder, between 3 and 7, depending upon your fitness level.

Bikini Tip

Take 3 deep, long breaths before you start to eat. This gives you time to relax and pay attention so you don't lapse into mindless eating habits.

to the end of your flow sequence. You can also try adding an extra 5 minutes of movement to your routine.

End with the *pranayama* of your choice.

WALKING: 45 Minutes to an Hour

Today all beginners should pick up the pace, progressing from 30 minutes to 45, and those who are more advanced should continue with the full hour. No matter how long your walk, be sure to move at a brisk pace and keep your heart rate up to receive the full benefits.

CIRCUIT TRAINING: CIRCUIT B

By now you're more familiar with the circuit moves. Keep your eye on the clock and your pace steady.

CORE STRENGTHENING: SERIES A

As you perform each exercise, sense how your torso muscles are strengthening, making your waist and belly slimmer and tighter with every rep.

TODAY'S MEAL PLAN

MORNING BURST: Hot water with lemon
BREAKFAST: Amaranth Cooked Cereal (page 207)
LUNCH: Black Bean Salad (page 216)
SNACK: 1 apple with 1 tsp. all-natural peanut butter

DINNER: Clear Chicken Soup with Lime & Avocado (page 230)
Steamed Fish with Ginger Sauce served over Soba Noodles (page 247)
DESSERT: Pineapple Poached in Orange Juice & Brown Sugar (page 255)

Ginger Muscle Rub

To energize and warm your sore muscles, grate a small piece of fresh ginger and mix it with a palmful of unscented body lotion. Massage into your skin for a deliciously fragrant experience. This tingling and moisturizing treat feels especially great on the feet! Many skin-care lines already boast ginger body lotions—and other products—so it's fine to use one of theirs as well.

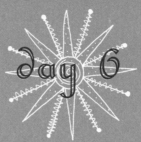

Day 6

The human body is the best picture of the human soul.
—*Ludwig Wittgenstein*

Journal Writing
Morning Meditation: Release and Let Go
Yoga: 15 minutes of Sun Salutations
Walking: 15 minutes to 1 hour at a brisk pace
Circuit Training: Circuit C

It's Day 6, so you are now a bona fide Bikini Bootcamper! You're getting used to new ways of eating and moving . . . maybe you're even having fun. You probably feel as if you're standing taller and straighter and you undoubtedly are. Your energy is beginning to soar, and you're starting to enjoy a different kind of body awareness as you sense your newly toned muscles working throughout your day.

TODAY'S INSPIRATION IS LETTING GO

Some of the bonds that we have are healthy, but many of our attachments are the result of routine, convenience, or insecurity, and they may not be adding to our happiness or fulfillment. Take this opportunity to think about the trappings of your life and whether or not your rela-

tionships, commitments, and other circumstances are working for you. If there are people or any other aspects of your life that drain rather than enrich you, now is the time to let them go. Realize that letting go is a conscious choice, and now is the time to make that choice. Part of letting go means forgiving, and while forgiveness does not mean condoning, it helps you grow and take control over negative emotions that can sabotage the healthy changes you're making.

JOURNAL WRITING

In today's journaling, begin to explore the idea of letting go of stressful or negative aspects of your life. Imagine a situation in which you hold a serious grievance against someone, and say, "I release you from my sadness, anger, and condemnation." Write it out in your journal—the situation and the release—to neutralize your negative emotions. You'll be amazed at how easy it is to let go of things once you admit them to yourself on paper.

MORNING MEDITATION:
Release and Let Go

Sit comfortably and begin to establish your breath as you connect your focus to each inhalation and exhalation. Recognize each moment, each breath. With each exhalation, give yourself permission to release and let go of that which does not serve you. With each inhalation, embrace the new, empty space you are creating for positive change.

YOGA: 15 Minutes
of Sun Salutations

BEGINNERS: Continue to move at a pace that challenges you, again, not concerning yourself with the number of Sun Salutations you complete, but rather continuing to explore the breath, the *asanas* (postures), and your body.

INTERMEDIATE AND ADVANCED: Increase the pace, but only to the point where you can maintain a connection to your breath and body. Mix the flow up by incorporating extra poses and more challenging lunge sequences. Add an extra 5 minutes to your Sun Salutation sequence if you can. Finish with the *pranayama* of your choice.

WALKING: 45 Minutes to 1 Hour

If you're already walking the full hour, try to up the cardio benefits and caloric burn by taking on more challenging terrain.

CIRCUIT TRAINING: CIRCUIT C

Remember: Keep your eye on the clock. Are you close to completing 2 circuits within 38 minutes yet?

TODAY'S MEAL PLAN

MORNING START: Hot water with lemon
BREAKFAST: Banana Smoothie (page 207)
LUNCH: Mango Chicken Salad (page 222)
SNACK: 10 whole almonds with raisins
DINNER: Black Bean Soup (page 225)
Fish Tacos in Lettuce "Tortillas" with Salsa Verde (page 244)
DESSERT: Fresh Blueberries with Mint (page 252)

Bikini Tip

Send your intention to whichever muscles you want to activate and tone during your walk—for example, to the area where your thigh meets your butt or to your upper arms. Studies have confirmed that focusing your intention on a particular body part while you exercise it actually increases its tone!

Bikini Tip

After your workout, give yourself a relaxing and energizing massage to keep your energy up during your day. How can you massage those hard-to-reach parts? It's easy. Simply grab a tennis ball or any kind of firm, inflatable ball and roll it along your muscles. Lie on the floor and balance yourself on top of the ball so you can guide it where you want it to go. Hamstrings should be rolled from hip to knee; glutes should be rolled upward, and you always want to roll *up* the side of the spine and neck to lengthen those muscles and improve posture. Another rule for arms and legs is to always roll *away* from the torso. You might not look graceful, but trust us, the results are amazing!

Papaya from the Playa

Papaya fruit is indigenous to tropical climates around the world, and it is often used in top-line facial masks to nourish and moisturize the skin. The enzymes in papaya exfoliate rough, dull-looking dead skin and fight free radicals. It's especially good for aging or oily skin, or for those with adult acne. Simply remove the peel and use a piece to scrub away dead skin cells on your face, and condition your skin with vitamins A and C. Or you can try our back-to-basics moisturizing mask (and save a little for a healthy snack!):

> 1 ripe papaya
>
> 1/4 cup of plain yogurt

1. Take a quarter of a papaya, cut it into pieces, and put it in a blender with the yogurt. Blend until smooth.
2. Gently massage the mixture into your clean face, neck, upper chest, and hands.
3. Set for 10 minutes, then rinse with warm water.

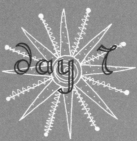

day 7

One day, when the wind is perfect, the sail just needs to open
and the world is full of beauty. Today is such a day.

—*Rumi*

Journal Writing
Morning Meditation: Choose your favorite
Yoga: 15 Minutes of Sun Salutations
Walking: 45 minutes to 1 hour at a brisk pace
Circuit Training: Circuit A
Core Strengthening: Series B

Congratulations! By the end of today you will have officially completed Week One of the program, so you deserve a reward. At Bikini Bootcamp, we reward our campers by turning physical exercise into local adventures—snorkeling in a *cenote* (freshwater cavern), kayaking in the open sea, or bicycling to Tulum's Mayan ruins. Why not reward yourself with an adventure in your area? Today, instead of your walk, grab a friend for an extra-long hike through a local park or up a nearby mountain. Treat yourself to a yoga, Pilates, skydiving, or belly dance class—whatever sparks your imagination. The only limitations are in your own mind! Whatever physical activity you choose, be sure to do it for at least one hour mini-

mum . . . the longer, the better, as long as you are enjoying yourself. Of course, if you prefer, you can always stick with your Bikini Bootcamp exercise program for the day.

TODAY'S INSPIRATION IS PLAYFULNESS

Now that you've almost completed one week of Bikini Bootcamp, take this opportunity to remember that this process, although challenging, is meant to be FUN! Today, tap into your inner child by trying something you have always wanted to try or participating in your favorite activity or pastime. Dance around your living room to your favorite music, take your BBC meals outdoors for a picnic, or stop by a park and take a few minutes to play on a swing or slide.

JOURNAL WRITING

Let your inner child write in your journal today, and allow her to write whatever she wants, unedited and uncensored. What did you treasure most about being young? How can you recapture some of those things and bring them back into your daily life? Allow this inner child to stay with you throughout the day . . . and the weeks to come!

MORNING MEDITATION

Choose your favorite meditation from the past six days.

YOGA: 15 Minutes
of Sun Salutations

BEGINNERS: Continue to move at a pace that challenges you, again, not concerning yourself with the number of Sun Salutations you complete, but rather continuing to explore the breath, the *asanas* (postures), and your body.

INTERMEDIATE AND ADVANCED: Increase the pace, but only to the point where you can maintain a connection to your breath and body. Mix the flow up by incorporating extra poses and add an extra 5 minutes to your Sun Salutation sequence if you can. Celebrate the end of your first week by adding an extra lunge sequence!

Complete your daily yoga session with your favorite *pranayama* from Chapter 3.

WALKING: 45 Minutes to 1 Hour

For those who can't plan an adventure, continue with your walking regimen of 45 minutes to 1 hour. If you are still struggling, don't worry—just increase your walking time as you are able.

CIRCUIT TRAINING: CIRCUIT A

By now this circuit should be familiar. Take note of how you feel when you do the exercises. Are the moves getting smoother, easier, more controlled? Are you less winded at the end of each set? If you feel ready, see if you can increase your three-pound weights to five—but never sacrifice your form.

CORE STRENGTHENING: SERIES B

After a week, most of our campers report that they can see amazing new definition in their abs and feel their posture changing. Are you standing taller? Carrying your shoulder bag with greater ease? Is your winter belly disappearing? Keep up the great work and before you know it, your torso will be toned and bikini-ready.

TODAY'S MEAL PLAN

MORNING BURST: Hot water with lemon
BREAKFAST: Scrambled Eggs with Spinach & Mushrooms (page 213)
LUNCH: Curried Spinach Salad with Grilled Fish, Papaya & Pumpkin Seeds (page 220)
SNACK: 2 tbsp. Guacamole (page 266) with carrot sticks
DINNER: Broccoli Soup (page 226) Chicken Stir-Fry over Chopped Napa Cabbage (page 242)
DESSERT: Grilled Banana with Caramel (page 254)

Treat Yourself

Buy yourself a gorgeous bunch of flowers today to congratulate yourself for a week well done! Let your nose guide you to the perfect kind of flowers and enjoy their soothing fragrance as it fills your home. For your spa treat, there won't be any do-it-yourself today: Schedule an hourlong massage or mani-pedi at your local spa!

MASSAGE oIL

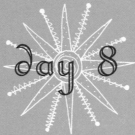

day 8

Life is either a daring adventure or nothing.
—*Helen Keller*

Journal Writing
Morning Meditation: Ten-Minute Breath
Yoga: 15 minutes of Sun Salutations
Walking: 45 minutes to 1 hour at a brisk pace
Circuit Training: Circuit B

Welcome to your second week at Bikini Bootcamp! This is a great time to take a moment to look back and congratulate yourself on all that you've achieved and the even greater things to come. Sense how you're already becoming more toned and shapely—you've likely already started to see new muscles—and congratulate yourself for raising the bar on your health and happiness. Keep eating right, moving right, and thinking right, and you will reach your goal before you know it. Your bikini body is just seven short days away!

TODAY'S INSPIRATION IS FAITH

Take a few minutes to think about the word "faith." In Western tradition, faith means to trust without seeing. The Sanskrit translation goes beyond this defi-

nition to mean trusting "from the heart." Today, even if you found the first week of the program incredibly challenging, believe with all your heart that you will complete the fourteen days successfully and get the results you want!

JOURNAL WRITING

Revisit your faith in today's journal writing. Ask yourself the following questions: Since I started Bikini Bootcamp, has my faith in my ability to accomplish my goals increased? Have I experienced more success on the program than I expected? Do I see myself as a stronger person today than I did one week ago? The answers to all those questions will hopefully be a resounding "Yes!" but if you're having doubts about your ability to stick with the plan for another week or see real changes in your body, now is the time to reaffirm your belief that your hard work will ultimately pay off. Put your determination and your faith into words on paper—just writing them down will make them stronger in your mind.

MORNING MEDITATION:
Ten-Minute Breath

Today we revisit the Ten-Minute Breath meditation from Day One. It's a perfect, simple way to center yourself and gear up for the week ahead.

1.   Find a comfortable seat, either on the floor or on a chair. Place your hands on your knees, palms facing down, to symbolize that all you need is within you already. If you are lying down, place your right hand on your heart, and your left hand on your belly.

2.   Allow your tongue to rest on the roof of your mouth and begin to establish your breathing by becoming aware of your breath.

3.   Now inhale and exhale through your nose. Allow your mind to follow your pattern of inhalations and exhalations, and do not hold your breath. Imagine energy flooding your body with each inhalation, and then let go of any impurities or negative thoughts with each exhalation. As thoughts come into your mind, acknowledge them and then let them go. Imagine these thoughts floating by you on a passing cloud, clearing your mind. Recognize that all that matters is this present moment symbolized by each breath.

YOGA: 15 Minutes
of Sun Salutations

BEGINNERS: Continue working for fluidity and building speed. If you feel ready, move on to the Intermediate Sun Salutation.

ADVANCED: Continue working to increase fluidity and repetitions, adding on an extra 5 minutes if you can. Try to hold each pose for up to five breaths. Add the additional poses as desired.

Finish with the *pranayama* of your choice.

WALKING: 45 Minutes to 1 Hour

You've now been walking daily for over a week, so you should be able to sense a difference in your level of aerobic fitness. Remember to keep your heart rate up for maximum benefits and caloric burn.

Bikini Tip
Walking has been known to stimulate creativity, so if it suits your schedule, plan your walk on your lunch hour or before a business meeting for added mental benefits.

CIRCUIT TRAINING: CIRCUIT B

Are you completing 2 rounds in 38 minutes yet? Don't worry, you soon will be! Keep up a steady, even pace.

TODAY'S MEAL PLAN

MORNING BURST: Hot water with lemon
BREAKFAST: Mango Madness Smoothie (page 211)
LUNCH: Soba Noodle Salad with Sesame Chicken (page 222)
SNACK: Cucumber sticks with lime and salt
DINNER: Sopa de Lima (page 233)
Grilled Fish with Radish, Cucumber, & Jicama Salad (page 245)
DESSERT: Baked Pear with Brown Sugar & Cinnamon (page 252)

Luscious Lips

Our homemade lip remedy is as good as any gloss—and much less expensive! Mix a pinch of sugar with 1 teaspoon of olive oil and gently massage on your lips for 2 minutes. This not only soothes chapped lips, it also helps prevent any additional chapping, leaving your lips soft and kissable.

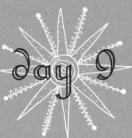

day 9

People often say that beauty is in the eye of the beholder, and I say that the most
liberating thing about beauty is that you are the beholder. This empowers us to find
beauty in places where others have not dared to look, including inside ourselves.

—*Salma Hayek*

Journal Writing
Morning Meditation: De-Stress
Yoga: 15 minutes of Sun Salutations
Walking: 1 hour at a brisk pace
Circuit Training: Circuit C
Core Strengthening: Series A

Hang in there! You know you're an inspiration to all of your friends. Maybe some of them have even signed on to your new lifestyle. Are you loving what you see in your mirror yet? How about those skinny jeans? Have you brought them out of the back of the closet yet? You're nearly there!

TODAY'S INSPIRATION
IS FLEXIBILITY

Flexibility breeds contentment. Life does not always go as planned, and one of its major challenges is learning how to deal with the obstacles that are placed in front of us. Today, work not only on your physical flexibility but your emotional flexibility as well. Changing our patterns and habits can be tough. But the more you open yourself to the brand-new precepts of Bikini Bootcamp, the more natural they will become.

JOURNAL WRITING

Envision a situation that requires you to be flexible. As you write, explore your possible choices of action in this scenario, aiming for greater and greater flexibility, until you arrive at the best possible choice and outcome. Sometimes our options become clearer more easily on the page than they do in our minds.

MORNING MEDITATION: De-Stress

Today we revisit the de-stress meditation to help you pinpoint exactly where you are holding tension so you can let it go. Freedom from stress helps breed a more flexible, go-with-the-flow attitude. So the next time you are stuck in traffic or waiting in line, or getting impatient with any other situation, find your breath and focus on it rather than on your frustrations.

1. Sit down somewhere comfortable and close your eyes. Take a few deep inhalations through your nose and exhale through your mouth.
2. Continuing to breathe deeply, focus on the top of your head and your forehead, sensing any tension and giving it permission to go.
3. Move progressively through the rest of your body, sensing any tension in each group of muscles and letting it go.
4. After you finish, take a quick inventory of any muscles still holding tension and let that tension go.

YOGA: 15 Minutes of Sun Salutations

BEGINNERS: Keep up the flow by moving through the poses as steadily as possible and increasing the rate. If you feel ready, move on to the Intermediate Sun Salutation.

ADVANCED: Continue working to increase fluidity and repetitions, adding on an extra 5 minutes if you can. Experiment with holding each posture for up to five breaths. Add additional poses as desired.

Top off your Sun Salutations with the *pranayama* of your choice.

WALKING: One Hour!

Now that you're a regular walker, you should be up to speed and capable of putting in a full hour. Even if you intersperse your brisk walking with a couple of intervals done at a slower pace, keep moving for the entire hour if you can. If you're still working hard to complete the 45 minutes, don't worry—if you continue to make walking your daily habit, you'll be logging an hour in no time. If you're already walking the full hour and would like an extra challenge, try wearing a weighted vest or taking on more hilly terrain.

CIRCUIT TRAINING: CIRCUIT C

Be sure to maintain an even pace, proper form, and keep your eye on the clock!

CORE STRENGTHENING: SERIES A

Form is everything in core strengthening, so take your time, even as the exercises become familiar. Remember, fewer repetitions performed well is better than more repetitions with incorrect form.

TODAY'S MEAL PLAN

MORNING BURST: Hot water with lemon
BREAKFAST: Banana Yogurt Parfait (page 208)

LUNCH: Fresh Spinach & Chickpea Salad with Tomatoes & Walnuts (page 221)
SNACK: 10 whole almonds with one tbsp. raisins

DINNER: Cauliflower Soup (page 229) Chicken Curry with Veggies on Whole-Grain Couscous (page 239)
DESSERT: Fresh mango

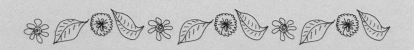

Blush Brush

Though it might sound unusual, brushing your skin with a dry body brush (available in health food stores and high-end cosmetic stores and pharmacies) is a great circulation stimulator and a wonderful way to get going in the morning and show the world your rosy hue. Before you take a long, steamy bath or shower, use a natural-bristle brush with a long handle to brush every part of your body, except your face and neck. Make long, sweeping strokes, always moving toward the heart: Brush from the hands to the shoulders, the feet up to the thighs, and the sides of the back toward the front of your torso. If you brush and then bathe, be sure to follow the hot bath or shower with a short blast of cold water to shake off any grogginess and close your pores.

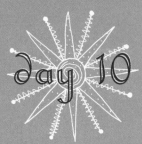

day 10

To tend unfailingly, unflinchingly, toward a goal is the secret to success.

—Anna Pavlova

Journal Writing
Morning Meditation: Tonglin
Yoga: 15 minutes of Sun Salutations
Walking: 1 hour at a brisk pace
Circuit Training: Circuit A

You're on the home stretch! Nearly there! By now, just like our Bikini Bootcampers, you're likely waking up each morning, bouncing out of bed, and heading straight for your mat to do your Sun Salutations. Your clothes are feeling looser, and your taste buds are also changing, so instead of craving a sugar or carb fix, you find yourself lusting for fresh pineapple. Indulge!

TODAY'S INSPIRATION IS GENEROSITY

Generosity means far more than monetary giving. A simple smile can brighten someone's entire day, not to mention your own. Take time today to give to someone else in the simplest of ways, whether it takes the form of a compliment, a thank-you, a smile, or helping an elderly person

cross the street. Your return will be tenfold, in terms of how you feel about yourself, because you'll know that you have enhanced someone else's day. And the better you feel about yourself, the easier it will be to keep up with these last few days of the regimen—because you know that no matter how hard the process might be, a fit and healthy body is what you deserve.

JOURNAL WRITING

In today's journaling, reflect on ways that you can be generous with others. Is there someone who needs a little more from you right now? Is there a way to give back to those around you? You should also reflect on how to be generous with yourself. Bikini Bootcamp is all about taking time for *you*—to look better, feel better, and put a spring in your step.

MORNING MEDITATION: Tonglin

As you learned on Day 3, the goal of this practice is to transform self-defeating thoughts into positive energy. If you've been hard on yourself because you haven't been progressing as quickly as you'd like, this meditation will help you see the changes you've made in a different light.

1. Come to a comfortable seated position or lie down, if necessary. Think of someone or something that needs your positive thoughts. This can be anything or anyone, even yourself if you need support.
2. Inhale through your nose, imagining that you are drawing in all the negativity, pain, and suffering that surround this person or situation. As you exhale, imagine that you are transforming all the negativity into peace, love, compassion, hope, and positive thoughts and energy for this person or situation.
3. Follow this breathing pattern for at least 5 breaths.

YOGA: 15 Minutes of Sun Salutations

Continue with your 15-minute Sun Salutation flows at the appropriate level for you. Be present and focused, challenging your body as much as you feel comfortable. The basics of the flows and the breathing should be easier by now. If you have yet to try the next level up or any of the extra *asanas,* now is the time to give it a shot.

WALKING: 1 Hour

If yesterday was your first day doing the full hour, how did it feel? Even if it wasn't easy, take pride in what you've achieved thus far. Soon that hour will pass in the blink of an eye! If you've been doing the full hour all along, be sure to keep challenging yourself, either by tackling a more difficult route or by walking at an even faster pace.

CIRCUIT TRAINING: CIRCUIT A

Keep it steady and keep your eye on the clock! Try to hit your timing target and do 2 circuits in 38 minutes.

TODAY'S MEAL PLAN

MORNING BURST: Hot water with lemon
BREAKFAST: Hard-Boiled Eggs with Salsa Mexicana (page 210)
LUNCH: Jicama, Black Bean, & Avocado Salad (page 221)
SNACK: 1 cup low-fat yogurt with 1 tbsp. raisins
DINNER: Butternut Squash Soup (page 227)
Amansala Salad with Grilled Fish & Ginger-Sesame Dressing (page 215)
DESSERT: Pineapple Frappé (page 255)

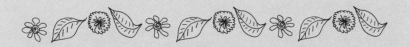

Reverse Relaxer

This rejuvenating ritual makes use of a restorative yoga pose and the healing properties of chamomile. Lie down in front of a wall and extend both legs up on it. Your buttocks should be up against the base of the wall with your legs perpendicular to your torso. Place chamomile tea bags that have been soaked a few moments in warm water over each eye to get rid of under-eye bags and make your eyes sparkle. Close your eyes and relax, allowing your blood and lymph to flow in a new way, for at least 5 minutes. This posture increases circulation, refreshes your entire body and brain, and helps counter the effects of gravity. You'll be standing taller before you know it!

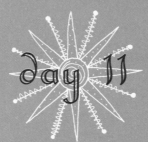

day 11

Without discipline, there is no life at all.
—*Katharine Hepburn*

Journal Writing
Morning Meditation: Walking Meditation
Yoga: 15 minutes of Sun Salutations
Walking: 1 hour at a brisk pace
Circuit Training: Circuit B
Core Strengthening: Series B

Look at all you've accomplished in just ten short days! Now take a quick peek into the near future: Just four more days and you'll be bikini-ready! Start planning a shopping spree, because you're going to want to flaunt your new slim and curvy shape. Pat yourself on the back and keep going!

TODAY'S INSPIRATION IS PATIENCE

Everything in life is a journey, a process, including the BBC lifestyle program. By now you should be well on your way to a bikini body, but don't look at your goals in this program as an all-or-nothing or success-or-failure matter. Instead, ask yourself if your actions are moving you in the right *direction*. Celebrate your successes and know that you are on your way!

JOURNAL WRITING

Allow your thoughts to come freely onto your paper as you ask yourself if you've been patient with yourself and your progress on this program. Give yourself the same patience and understanding that you would your best friend, and be happy with your success so far.

MORNING MEDITATION:
Walking Meditation

Practice the following meditation during your walk today. Walk in silence—no music, no friend, no cell phone—and allow your walk to become a chance to quiet the constant commentary that runs through your mind. Be mindful of your breath, the sounds and sights around you. If you typically walk indoors on a treadmill, take your walk outside, if weather permits, and enjoy all of nature's little gifts.

During the cooldown phase of your walk, do a moving meditation by slowing your pace and noticing your surroundings, counting your footsteps, or repeating a phrase or word that calms you—in other words, a mantra. Our campers like to repeat "calm," "peace," "relax," or the traditional yogic mantra, the sound of "Om." Lengthen your inhalations and exhalations, and concentrate on the rhythm of your movement.

YOGA: 15 Minutes
of Sun Salutations

Keep up a good pace, remembering to breathe properly and make your movements steady. No matter what your level, now is a good time to add 5 minutes to your practice (or even more if you like!). Have fun by adding some of the extra *asanas* on pages 103–106 to the end of your flow sequence.

WALKING: 1 Hour

Even if it's hard, keep pushing for the full hour! If you've been doing the full hour

all along, try some basic interval training, alternating 5 minutes of jogging with 10 minutes of brisk walking—or jogging for however long you feel comfortable.

CIRCUIT TRAINING: CIRCUIT B

By now, you should be completing 2 circuits in 38 minutes. If not, don't worry; just keep up your best pace and you'll get there soon enough!

CORE STRENGTHENING: SERIES B

Keep in mind: Form is everything. Feel your waist tightening and slimming!

TODAY'S MEAL PLAN

MORNING BURST: Hot water with lemon
BREAKFAST: Amaranth Cooked Cereal (page 207)
LUNCH: Crunchy Chicken Salad with Raisins & Apples (page 219)
SNACK: 2 cups fresh watermelon
DINNER: Gazpacho (page 230) Chicken Enchiladas with Tomato-Cilantro Sauce & Black Bean Puree (page 240)
DESSERT: Grilled Banana with Caramel (page 254)

Bikini Tip

If you're a new mom who wants to get back in shape, you can plunk baby in the stroller and set out for your walk. Boost the cardio value of your walk by adding 30 seconds of lunges every 2 minutes. Stand by the side of your stroller with your hand grasping the center of the handle. Then push forward as you do walking lunges. You can also do the walking lunge without a stroller—or children!

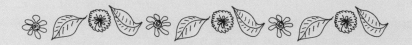

Jasmine Skin and Eye Calmer

Used as a facial steam or as a bath essence, this Far East delight soothes skin in a wonderfully fragrant way. When applied as a compress, it soothes tired and irritated eyes (and is said to spark libidos!). Simply boil water and pour into a bowl over jasmine flowers (available at Asian and health food stores) and prepare them as you would a tea, steeping for 5 minutes. If you cannot find jasmine flowers, jasmine tea bags will do just as well. To use as a steam, lean over the bowl and cover your head with a towel to trap the steam. Inhale for 5 minutes. Or, soak a wash-cloth in the fragrant water and apply it to your eyes as a warm compress.

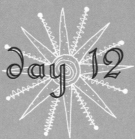

day 12

Miracles surround us at every turn if we sharpen our perception of them.

—*Willa Cather*

Journal Writing
Morning Meditation: Picture a beautiful place
Yoga: 15 minutes of Sun Salutations
Walking: 1 hour at a brisk pace
Circuit Training: Circuit C

We're excited—and we hope you are, too! It's been challenging, and your body may still have a few sore muscles, but by now you're likely convinced that it's all been worth it. In fact, you may not want to stop after two weeks! Don't worry: We've laid out a maintenance plan in Part IV that ensures you'll stay slim, toned, and healthy all your life. And if you want to continue shedding pounds, we tell you how to do that, too.

TODAY'S INSPIRATION IS PASSION

Think of something that brings you joy. Something that makes your heart smile and your soul sing. It may be a person, a pet, a hobby, or an interest. Now ask yourself how much time you actually allow yourself to cultivate and explore this passion. Staying active with hobbies and interests outside our daily routine not only inspires us, it also makes us feel alive. Try to approach your BBC regimen today with equal passion and know that you are doing wonders for your body and well-being!

JOURNAL WRITING

Explore your passions in your journaling today. Think "out of the box"—your only limitation is your mind. After you've written down five things you feel passionate about, go back and write down two "doable" steps toward exploring these passions. If you wrote down "ballerina," it may be a bit too late to join the New York City Ballet, but it's never too late to take ballet lessons or go to the ballet on a regular basis. There are always ways to get closer to the people, things, and activities you love if you think creatively. Hopefully your commitment to the BBC program and the great results you're already experiencing have proven that, with focus, you can do anything!

MORNING MEDITATION:
Picture a Beautiful Place

This meditation is a treat because it shows the power of your imagination. It can take you anywhere, even on a quickie tropical escape.

1. Get comfortable either sitting on a chair or cross-legged on the floor, and close your eyes.

2. Begin by breathing rhythmically as you inhale fresh oxygen through your nose and exhale tension through your mouth. Imagine any lingering negativity dissipating into nothing as it leaves your body.

3. Now picture a beautiful place, like the beach at Tulum. Smell the sea air, feel how the sun warms your skin, and let this image guide your body in letting go more and more.

4. Clench your toes and release them a few times, letting them relax. Move up through your body, tightening and releasing each muscle group. You're still on the beach, feeling the breeze, hearing the palm trees rustle, and sensing the sand beneath your feet.

5. After you've relaxed your entire body, come out of your relaxed state gradually by wiggling your toes and fingers, then giving yourself a good stretch.

YOGA: 15 Minutes
of Sun Salutations

Perform your Sun Salutations today with presence, fluidity, and enjoyment. Do your flow at a brisk pace and incorporate more challenging postures from the level above you, if you can. Try to add on an extra 5 or 10 minutes—hopefully the flows will feel so good you won't want to stop! Remember to finish with the *pranayama* of your choice.

WALKING: 1 Hour

Since ancient times, walking has been a part of many rites of passage. So as you begin winding down the program, let your daily walk not only help you lose weight and tone those thighs, but also firm up your determination to finish your own rite of passage—completing the Bikini Bootcamp program and holding on to your gains for the rest of your life!

CIRCUIT TRAINING: CIRCUIT C

Are we having fun yet? Our campers love going through the circuits, and by now you should be loving it, too! Feel those muscles work and enjoy the satisfaction that comes from a good sweat.

TODAY'S MEAL PLAN

MORNING BURST: Hot water with lemon

BREAKFAST: Pineapple Swirl (page 212)

LUNCH: Couscous Salad with Mint, Raisins & Almonds (page 218)

SNACK: Carrot sticks with Hummus (page 266)

DINNER: Lentil Soup (page 231) Vegetable Fajitas with Black Beans, Guacamole, & Salsa Mexicana (page 249)

DESSERT: Fresh Mango with Shredded Coconut (page 253)

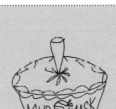

Tomato Face Mask

(NOT RECOMMENDED FOR SENSITIVE SKIN)

Tomatoes as a skin refresher—who knew? Believe it or not, the acids in tomatoes are great for getting rid of blackheads and will brighten dull skin by gently loosening surface cells. So they're not just delicious, they beautify as well.

1 ripe, medium-sized tomato

1 teaspoon of purifying clay mask (any brand will do)

Puree the tomato and then add the clay mask. Mix well and apply to face, neck, upper chest, and hands. Leave on for 10 to 15 minutes. Rinse well with warm water.

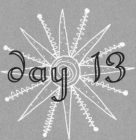

day 13

Success is liking yourself, liking what you do, and liking how you do it.
—*Maya Angelou*

Journal Writing
Morning Meditation: Mantras
Yoga: 15 minutes of Sun Salutations
Walking: 1 hour at a brisk pace
Circuit Training: Circuit A
Core Strengthening: Series A

The end is in sight, but it's really just the beginning! You've worked your butt off . . . literally! Be proud of all you've accomplished and know that you've done even more than whittle your shape down to bikini-perfect size. You've embarked on a new lifestyle that will keep you looking and feeling great long after these two weeks are over!

TODAY'S INSPIRATION IS SERENITY

Amidst our many responsibilities, e-mails, cell phones, offices, and even our family and friends, it is often rare to find moments of serenity. The challenge in today's world is to find serenity within, to discover the calm within the storm of your daily life. Use the tools you have acquired throughout the past two weeks, such as the meditations and *pranayamas,* to assist you in tapping into your own serenity today.

JOURNAL WRITING

What makes you feel serene? It might be a special person or place, a memory or moment, a feeling, a song, or an activity. Whatever it is, take some time today to write about it. See if you can find a way to make serenity a greater presence in your life.

MORNING MEDITATION: Mantras

Mantras are sounds, words, or phrases that calm us and harmonize our energy. We focus on repeating a mantra during meditation in order to still our minds of constant chatter. You can chant "Om" (the universal sacred sound) or some other personal mantra ("one," "love," "peace," or "calm") or phrases such as "let go," or any other brief, prayerful phrase that has significance for you and quiets your mind. In yoga, we traditionally begin and end our practice with everyone chanting "Om" on an exhalation. If a different thought crosses your mind during meditation, don't panic. Simply observe it, let it go, and return to repeating your mantra.

1. Sit down comfortably and close your eyes.
2. Start by breathing deeply and regularly, inhaling through your nose and exhaling out of your mouth.
3. Relax your muscles from head to toe.
4. Begin repeating your mantra as you breathe. Passively disregard all other thoughts that come to your mind and just keep returning to repetition of your mantra. Continue this way for 5 minutes.

YOGA: 15 Minutes of Sun Salutations

If you haven't moved on to the next level, now is the time to go for it. If you don't feel ready, don't worry; just continue practicing your 15-minute (or more) Sun Salutation flow in a steady, brisk rhythm and move on as you are able. Choose a *pranayama* to top off your routine.

WALKING: 1 Hour

Take the scenic route today and treat yourself to a change from your usual walking routine.

CIRCUIT TRAINING: CIRCUIT A

Are you addicted yet? Have your individual circuit stations become a permanent part of your living room decor? Keep going—there's only one more day!

CORE STRENGTHENING: SERIES A

Enjoy the sensation of your muscles tautening and flattening, and your waist getting tinier and tinier!

TODAY'S MEAL PLAN

MORNING BURST: Hot water with lemon

Bikini Tip: Tap Away Tension
If you still feel tense, lightly tap your scalp with your knuckles for 20 seconds as you breathe slowly and deeply. This softens tense muscles and boosts energy.

BREAKFAST: Ginger Pineapple Smoothie (page 210)
LUNCH: Asian Chicken Lettuce Wraps with Crushed Peanuts (page 215)
SNACK: Spicy Black Bean Dip with carrot sticks (page 268)

DINNER: Spicy Mexican Vegetable Soup (page 234)
Grilled Fish with Mango Salsa (page 245)
DESSERT: Homemade Blueberry Sorbet (page 254)

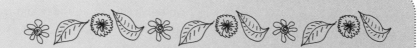

Vita Carrot Mask

Carrots are incredibly rich in vitamin A, which promises anti-aging activity when applied topically to the skin. This sweet-smelling mask is good for even the most sensitive skin. The oils can be found in most health food stores.

> 1 large carrot, peeled and chopped fine
>
> 1 tbsp. sweet almond oil
>
> 5 drops jasmine essential oil (optional)

1. Puree the carrot in a blender or food processor and strain off the juice. Blend the pulp with sweet almond oil and add jasmine essential oil drop by drop.

2. Mix it well and apply the pulp to a freshly cleansed face, avoiding the eye and mouth area. Allow the mask to set for 15 minutes. Rinse well with warm water and apply moisturizer as usual.

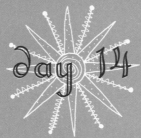

day 14

Look at a day when you are supremely satisfied at the end. It's not a day when you lounge around doing nothing; it's when you had everything to do, and you've done it.

—*Margaret Thatcher*

Journal Writing
Morning Meditation: Golden Light
Yoga: 15 minutes of Sun Salutations
Walking: 1 hour at a brisk pace
Circuit Training: Circuit B

Congratulations! Welcome to the last day of Bikini Bootcamp and the rest of your new life. Okay, it was tough, but wasn't it worth it? You've got new, glowing skin, a healthier approach to food, and a taut, slim bikini body! Give it all you've got today, and know that it's not over! In fact, BBC never ends, and you wouldn't want it to end anyway, would you? You want that bikini body forever, right? Our Bikini Bootcamp Lifestyle Plan in Part IV will ensure that this happens.

TODAY'S INSPIRATION IS CELEBRATE

Look back on all you have experienced, explored, and accomplished over the past two weeks. Now look forward to limitless possibilities for your health, fitness, and fun in the future. There is no end to this process; the fun has just begun! We'll show you how to keep your bikini body year-round with the maintenance plan in Part IV.

JOURNAL WRITING

Today's journaling is all about your achievements. Note all your successes from the past two weeks in today's entry and take a moment to recognize how they've made you feel. You can also take this moment to outline your goals for the future. We hope you'll be inspired to stick with the BBC program, and daily journaling will help keep you on the right track.

MORNING MEDITATION:
Golden Light

This meditation not only calms and energizes, it also gives you a powerful sense of connection to the Source (or however you define the larger workings of the universe).

1. Sit down comfortably and close your eyes.
2. Inhale and exhale deeply, and let your body find your breath. Now envision a stream of sparkling golden light flowing freely through your body, starting from the tip of your toes and moving all the way up to the top of your head.
3. Continue breathing as you imagine the light moving through your body and creating harmony and health wherever it goes.

YOGA: 15 Minutes
of Sun Salutations

The more you practice your Sun Salutations, the better—even after BBC is over—in fact, every day is ideal. Today, take your yoga practice outdoors if possible, so you can breathe the fresh air and enjoy the tranquility of nature as you bend, stretch, and twist. Don't worry if you're still in beginner mode; yoga is not a competitive sport. Keep up your practice and you'll naturally move up to a more advanced level over time. Always remember to finish with one of the *pranayamas* from Chapter 3.

WALKING: 1 Hour

Hopefully, just about everyone should be walking the full hour at this point. If this is not the case for you, don't worry. You'll get there! This may be the last day of your Bikini Bootcamp program, but walking is a habit you'll want to keep for the rest of your life. No matter the season, always rejoice that you are able to move freely out in the world!

CIRCUIT TRAINING: CIRCUIT B

We know you're just zipping through, clocking your progress and having the time of your life, right? After today, you can keep your bikini body by doing circuit training three times a week. Our BBC circuits are so effective that most of our campers wind up doing them long after they leave our sunny shores.

TODAY'S MEAL PLAN

MORNING BURST: Hot water with lemon
BREAKFAST: Fruit Bowl with Almonds (page 209)
LUNCH: Amansala Salad with Grilled Chicken & Ginger-Sesame Dressing (page 215)
SNACK: Cucumber sticks and 2 tbsp. Guacamole (page 266)
DINNER: Zucchini Soup (page 237) Steamed Fish with Tomatoes, Peppers, & Onions (page 248)
DESSERT: Whole-Grain Apple Crisp (page 256)

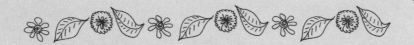

Oatmeal-Rose Skin Restoring Bath

A relaxing bath at the end of your final BBC day is a perfect opportunity not only to reward yourself, but also to restore moisture to your skin and exfoliate dead cells. With this final treatment, you'll officially be ready for the beach!

1. Mix 3 parts ground oatmeal (grind it in your blender) and 1 part fresh or dried rose petals in a small bowl.
2. Pour a handful of the mixture into a nylon stocking and tie off the top. Place it in your bath as it fills.

You can also exfoliate dead cells by gently rubbing a handful of sea salt over your skin while you're in the bath. Use a bath brush or loofah for hard-to-reach places. If your skin tends to be dry, add 1 teaspoon of olive oil or 1/2 cup of whole milk to the bathwater.

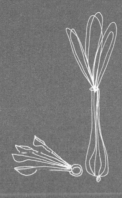

PART III

The Cookbook

You don't have to cook fancy or complicated
masterpieces—just good food from fresh ingredients.
—Julia Child

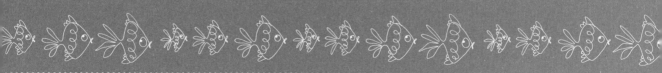

At Bikini Bootcamp,

we believe that eating should always be a pleasure, and our recipes are designed not only to help you lose weight, but also to genuinely enjoy food and its preparation. If you're the kind of girl who subsists on coffee and sandwiches from the deli, the next two weeks will open the door to a whole new world of culinary delights. We're just like you, and we know that you don't have hours to spend preparing food every day—there are jobs, families, and social obligations, not to mention all those BBC workouts to contend with! So our goal has been to create an eating plan that delivers delicious, nutritious, low-calorie food in keeping with our back-to-basics philosophy via recipes that are straightforward and incredibly easy to whip up in a short time.

Before you dive into the recipes themselves, take a look at the overview that follows of the most-used BBC ingredients, as well as our lists of preparation tips and possible substitutions to help you plan for the weeks ahead. You'll also find separate shopping lists for Weeks One and Two, a complete list of healthy snacks, and a list of the cooking staples that you'll want to have in your pantry at all times.

We recommend that you start the two-week program on a Monday, so you'll have the weekend to shop for groceries and prepare for the coming week by chopping vegetables, making soups and sides, and mixing dressings in advance.

What's Cooking?

No matter how much of a cook you are, or how versatile your eating habits, there will likely be a few ingredients in our recipes that will be gracing your table for the first time. Some—like jicama, papaya, and black beans—are typical Mexican and Latin American fare. Others—like curry or soba noodles—come from different Asian cuisines and are a result of Melissa's years as a chef in Japan. Each food you'll find on the BBC menus plays a specific role in your weight-loss program and brings its own unique health benefits to the mix. Here are some of our most commonly used ingredients and a few words about how and why we use them.

- **Almonds.** A terrific, tasty source of protein, almonds are a high-fat food that's actually good for you. Studies show that their healthy fats

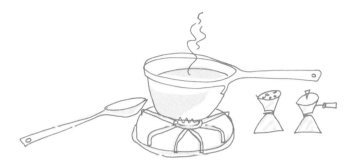

lower bad cholesterol and reduce the risk of heart disease; they also allow your body to absorb essential nutrients found in other foods. At Amansala, we top off breakfasts, salads, and even desserts with this sweet yet savory nut; many of our daily snacks also include almonds for a metabolism-boosting protein fix. It only takes a few to get the nutrition you need!

• **Amaranth.** A grain indigenous to Mexico, amaranth is high in both protein and fiber and boasts three times the iron and fiber content of wheat, and two times the calcium content of milk. It is easy on the digestive tract and is often given to those recovering from an illness. These days you can buy amaranth and amaranth-based cereals at many regular supermarkets as well as at whole food and health food stores. If you've never tried it, the flavor may seem a bit unusual at first, but you will quickly develop a taste for it and likely come to crave it over blander grains like wheat.

• **Avocado.** Avocados may not be considered a low-calorie or low-fat food, but they contain the healthy fats you need to absorb and process essential vitamins and minerals, keep your energy levels up, and maintain healthy, glowing skin. You'll eat plenty of this yummy, quintessentially Mexican food throughout the program in our salads, guacamole, and more.

When buying avocados, keep in mind that you want to eat them when they are soft but not mushy. A hard avocado will take several days to ripen and should not be kept in the refrigerator.

···

- **Black Beans.** Black beans are a delicious staple of the Mexican diet, and they are full of B vitamins and fiber; plus, they are an excellent source of protein. We have many tasty uses for them throughout our meal plans—in salads, on their own, or as a side dish served with our famous Chicken Fajita recipe. Our recipes allow you to use canned beans, as dried beans are time-consuming to prepare from scratch. However, we've included two versions of our Basic Black Beans recipe on page 265—one that shows you how to prepare dried beans in the traditional way, and a faster method using canned.
- **Blueberries.** Bursting with flavor and very low in calories, blueberries are considered a "superfood" because they provide countless essential nutrients, including vitamin C, and pack a powerful antioxidant punch. Researchers at Tufts recently concluded that blueberries rated highest among all fruits in their ability to destroy disease-causing free radicals! While they are difficult to find in Mexico, we take advantage of them whenever we can.
- **Cabbage.** A cruciferous vegetable (along with broccoli, cauliflower, and kale), cabbage not only delivers a hefty dose of fiber to help you feel full, it also provides high doses of vitamins K and C and acts as a natural detoxifier. The phytonutrients in cabbage actually signal your genes to produce enzymes involved in detoxification, optimizing your cells' ability to rid themselves of free radicals and toxins—all of which supports your goals of getting your body and your metabolism to function in high gear.
- **Chicken.** Chicken is an excellent source of lean protein, providing 67.6 percent of the recommended daily allowance in just 4 ounces. Protein keeps your metabolism supercharged throughout the day, preventing blood sugar crashes between meals and giving you the building blocks you need to build new muscle through your workouts. You want to avoid antibiotic- and hormone-laced meats as much as you can, so buy organic, free-range chicken whenever possible.

- **Chickpeas (Garbanzo Beans).** Used in salads, hummus, and soups, chickpeas are a valuable source of protein that add zing to any dish with their appealing, nutty flavor. You can buy fresh hummus at your local Mediterranean food store or make your own, using our recipe on page 266. Just steer clear of those preprepared brands sold in supermarkets, as they are often loaded with sugars and additives; be sure to check labels.
- **Curry.** Curry powder, a readily available Western blend of spices designed to approximate Indian spice blends, typically contains turmeric, coriander, chilis, cumin, mustard, ginger, fenugreek, garlic, cloves, salt, and any number of other spices. The spice with the most noted health benefits is turmeric, which gives curry powder its yellow color, aids digestion, helps fight infection, and reduces the risk of heart disease. It has also been linked to a lower incidence of Alzheimer's. If you've never tried curry, or don't find Indian food appealing, we urge you to give the recipes here a chance. Our curried salad dressing and other dishes are very mild and are made with standard, brand-name curry powder off the spice rack at your supermarket. No need for anything more exotic!
- **Fish.** We love fish because it is not only in keeping with Bikini Bootcamp's oceanfront, back-to-basics atmosphere, it's also an excellent source of lean protein and rich in omega-3 fatty acids (essential fatty acids that have anti-inflammatory benefits and may reduce the risk of heart disease). When preparing the recipes, opt for any kind of white, flaky fish: halibut, sea bass, grouper, snapper, orange roughy, cod, trout, tilapia, or flounder are all great choices. Fish that is fresh and local to your area is a good option as well.
- **Flax Seeds.** Flax seeds are a valuable source of fiber and omega-3 fatty acids. They are delicious and nutty in flavor and can be added to any dish; sprinkle them over salads or over yogurt, or add them to smoothies for a healthy boost.
- **Fruit.** Fruit is often referred to as "nature's candy," and we understand why—it's tasty, sweet, and full of essential vitamins and minerals. Feel free to experiment with any kinds of fruit you like, especially those that are in season or grown locally. Our recipes make use of tropical fruits that are readily available in Tulum, but other fruits like raspberries, strawberries, cherries, peaches, and pears

work just as well. If certain fruits are not available in your area—or if, like blueberries, they become expensive during the winter—frozen fruits are okay to use as a substitute, provided they do not have any added sugars.

- **Garlic.** In addition to the wonderful flavor it brings to many dishes, garlic is a known immune-booster with antiviral and antibacterial properties. It also lowers cholesterol and may reduce the risk of cardiovascular disease. On the BBC meal plans, you'll discover a variety of new, delicious ways to enjoy garlic beyond the standard Italian-style, refined-carb-laden pizzas and pastas. It also makes a terrific substitute for salt.

Bikini Tip ....

Love salt? Try spicing up your food with a bit of garlic, ginger, or fresh herbs. Too much salt leads to water retention and an energy slump; it also increases your risk of high blood pressure and heart disease.

....

- **Ginger.** Asian societies have long known about the health benefits of ginger. In addition to bringing its zesty flavor to many BBC meals, this versatile root aids digestion, lowers blood pressure, and is a good circulatory stimulant. Whether tickling your taste buds or your skin (as in our Ginger Muscle Rub on page 156), fresh ginger is invigorating and a terrific addition to your cooking repertoire.
- **Jicama.** Jicama is a popular Latin American root vegetable with a mild taste and high water content so it fills you up fast. A rich source of potassium and fiber, it figures in many of our salads and snacks. If you can't find it in your local store, substitute carrots or celery instead.
- **Lemons and Limes.** Lemons and limes are citrus powerhouses that bring out the flavor in any food. They also contain high levels of vitamin C as well as unique flavonoid compounds that have antioxidant, anticancer, and even antibacterial properties. These refreshing, tangy fruits are a staple of BBC dressings, marinades, salads, dinners, and even some desserts, so be sure you stock up anytime you're at the store. For a thirst-quenching, antioxidant blast, try our signature Ginger Limeade recipe on page 270. Or add a squeeze of lemon or lime to your water throughout the day.

To get the most juice out of lemons and limes, roll them back and forth on the counter a few times before cutting, pressing down with your palm. Then cut them open as desired and squeeze.

- **Mango.** Mangoes are plentiful in Mexico and becoming more and more available in the United States. Rich in vitamin C, they are also an excellent source of beta-carotene, which your body can convert to vitamin A. If you can't find mangoes, feel free to substitute fresh oranges in any of the recipes.
- **Olive Oil.** Studies have shown that olive oil offers protection against heart disease and lowers bad cholesterol due to its antioxidant properties and high content of healthy, monounsaturated fats. We recommend that you use extra virgin, or cold-pressed, olive oil in all our recipes, which contains higher levels of antioxidants, particularly vitamin E, because it is less processed.
- **Papaya.** Once considered quite exotic, papayas can now be found in most U.S. grocery stores, and we love to incorporate this classic tropical fruit into our dishes. Papayas are a great source of vitamins C and A, the B vitamins, flavonoids, and fiber, and they have antioxidant properties as well.

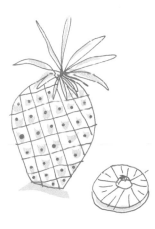

Many people don't like the taste of papaya, but there's an easy way to give it better flavor. Simply drizzle a little fresh lime juice on your papaya and see how it transforms the taste!

- **Pineapple.** At Amansala we serve pineapple almost every day, and even if our guests rarely have it at home, they devour this juicy fruit here whenever they can. Pineapple not only aids digestion, ensuring that you absorb vitamins and nutrients from other foods, but it is also a terrific source of fiber and vitamin C.
- **Pumpkin Seeds.** Indigenous to the Mayan region of Mexico, pumpkin seeds are rich in amino acids and provide high amounts of protein, monounsaturated (healthy) fats, magnesium, and iron. Sprinkling them over any of the BBC salads is an easy way to add extra vitamins and minerals to your meal.
- **Sesame Seeds.** Sesame seeds may be the earliest condiment known to man, dating back to 1600 B.C.! The nutty taste and satisfying crunch make them a favorite addition to Asian dishes, and they top many of the meals on the BBC program. They are high in copper, calcium, and magnesium, and also contain two unique substances—sesamin and sesamolin—that have cholesterol-lowering effects and protect the liver from oxidative damage. We use toasted rather than regular sesame seeds throughout our recipes, as toasting releases their nutty flavor.
- **Spinach.** Calorie for calorie, green, leafy vegetables like spinach provide more nutrients than any other food. They're also an excellent source of fiber to fill you up—and as such, spinach, which is high in iron and antioxidants, plays a role in many of our meals. You'll find countless new ways to enjoy this tasty green, starting with our signature Amansala Salad. In Mexico we use chaya, which is similar to spinach, so if you feel like a little Latin flavor, seek out some chaya at a gourmet market near you.

Bikini Tip
Anytime you prepare fresh spinach, either for cooking or for salads, be sure to wash the leaves thoroughly to remove sand, and cut off the stems.

- **Tomatoes.** A juicy, ripe tomato just might be the world's most perfect food, and we make plenty of use of these sumptuous fruits throughout our plan, most notably in our traditional Mexican Salsa. Tomatoes are high in vitamins A and C, and contain lycopene, a powerful antioxidant that directly counteracts the aging effects of sun exposure. Perfect for your beach prep!
- **Whole Grains.** With so many new products on the market, whole grains do not have to be tasteless or intimidating. Our meal plan incorporates whole-wheat couscous, soba noodles, amaranth, and flax seeds (see above); bulgar wheat and brown rice are good substitutes as well.
- **Yogurt.** On the BBC meal plan, the yogurt you eat should always be low-fat plain or vanilla, and organic if possible. As we mentioned in Chapter 5, dairy products are a great source of vitamins A, D, and all the B vitamins. They are also an excellent source of calcium, which recent studies show may play a role in weight loss, as it boosts your metabolism. If you don't like yogurt, substitute nonfat milk instead.

A Word about Sweeteners

At Bikini Bootcamp we sweeten all of our drinks, including coffee and tea, with stevia, a South American shrub whose leaves have been used for centuries by native peoples as a natural sweetener. It is virtually calorie-free, and it is hundreds of times sweeter than table sugar, so a little goes a long way. Stevia does not significantly alter blood sugar levels and is thus attractive to diabetics. It can be found in health food stores.

If you are unable to find stevia, honey will also work well as a natural sweetener. But since honey has calories, it should be limited to no more than 2 tbsp. a day.

We do not recommend using any kind of artificial sweetener, as the number one rule of BBC eating is NATURAL! While the jury's still out on what the long-term health effects of artificial sweeteners may be, the safest, according to the Center for Science in the Public Interest, is Splenda.

Substitutions

If you have a food allergy or just really, really do not like some of the foods in the recipes that follow, there are plenty of easy substitutions you can make:

- If you do not eat chicken or fish, it is important that you substitute beans or tofu, as you will need the protein boost throughout the day. We do not use tofu at Amansala, as it is not easily found in Mexico, but it can be prepared in the same manner as chicken or fish and absorbs whatever flavor it is cooked with.
- When preparing the soups, you can swap the low-sodium chicken broth for a low-sodium vegetable broth to create a vegetarian version.
- If you do not like or cannot eat dairy, substitute low-fat soy milk or soy yogurt instead.
- If you cannot find mango, or it's too expensive, substitute fresh oranges instead.
- If you cannot find jicama, try cucumber or celery as an alternative.
- If you do not like cilantro, substitute fresh basil.
- If you can't find amaranth cooked cereal, substitute a high-fiber, 9- or 7-grain cold breakfast cereal such as Kashi, with at least 4 grams of fiber per serving.
- When it comes to your breakfast smoothies, we encourage you to mix up the fruits involved depending on what you have in your refrigerator: mango-banana, apple-blueberry, and strawberry-pineapple are all great combinations.
- You can substitute frozen fruit for fresh as long as there is no added sugar.
- For your afternoon snack or an emergency cravings fix, choose any one of the snacks found on the list below. These foods fill you up quickly with healthy, high-quality calories, so you won't need to worry about sabotaging your weight-loss program.

The Bikini Bootcamp Snack List

Anytime you feel hungry, simply reach for one of the healthy snacks listed below. These foods are packed with nutritional value, and even though they do contain calories, their high fiber content will fill you up more quickly than other kinds of snacks—thus ensuring that you eat less. One serving should do the trick.

Fruits: *Apples:* satisfy your need to crunch.
Peaches, plums, and pears: will curb a sugar craving in a hurry.
Watermelon: fills you up fast due to its high water content.
Pineapple: loaded with digestive enzymes to help you absorb vital nutrients.
Oranges and tangerines: a great vitamin C boost, especially during flu season!
Bananas: while a bit higher in calories, they provide a quick burst of natural sugar and will fuel your endurance before a workout.
Grapes: for a real treat, freeze them. They are perfect for a hot summer day!
Raisins: These make for a delicious snack that will satisfy your sweet tooth. Have 1–2 tbsp., and make sure there's no added sugar.
Fresh fruit blend: Combine 1 cup fruit, 1 cup ice, and a dash of sweetener in your blender. Makes a healthy version of an Italian ice!

Vegetables: *Carrot, celery, or cucumber sticks:* with salsa.
Jicama sticks: try these with a squeeze of lime juice and a dusting of chili powder for a Mexican kick. Yum!
Edamame: These Japanese-style soybeans offer a protein boost. Buy them frozen at your local supermarket or at a whole foods or Asian foods store.

Air-popped popcorn: A great natural source of fiber and only 100 calories a "pop"! The microwave kind is fine, so long as it's without butter (look for brands that have a fiber content of 4 grams or more per serving). Opt for a salt-free variety, and add your own flavoring with a dash of chili powder or cinnamon.

High-fiber crackers: One to three high-fiber crackers (4 grams or more per serving), such as Ak-Mak crackers, will satisfy your hunger.

Nuts: Almonds and walnuts make terrific healthy snacks that offer fiber, healthy fats, and extra protein if you're dragging. A BBC favorite combines walnuts and raisins: Mix 10 whole nuts with 1 tbsp. of raisins for a sweet, nutty treat that has wonderfully complementary flavors.

Yogurt: 1 cup of low-fat plain or vanilla yogurt will do the trick. Add 1 tbsp. of raisins or fresh fruit for variety.

Herbal teas: Iced or hot with a touch of sweetener will fill you up and satisfy your sweet tooth. Try our recipes in the beverage section on page 269.

Preparation Tips

As you get ready for your two-week kick-start, here are some suggestions to make your kitchen life as easy as possible. A little planning at the beginning of the week or the night before can make a big difference in how you cook—and thus in how you eat. Spending less time over the cutting board or stove means more time to relax and enjoy your food, and it frees up time for workouts, journaling, and other components of the BBC program.

Portions

All of our dinner and dessert recipes are designed to serve two, so if you're dining solo, simply cut the recipe amounts in half. Or, make the full recipe and save one portion for another meal later in the week. All of the lunches are interchangeable, as are the dinners, so feel free to mix and match depending on your tastes. Our breakfasts, lunches, and snacks serve one, so you can easily double or quadruple the amounts to suit your needs.

Our soup recipes, however, all serve four. This is intended to make your life easier. As we said in Chapter 5, when it comes to soups, we recognize that you may not have time to be boiling up a batch of soup every day from scratch. Therefore, unless you're serving dinner for four every night, we recommend that you flip through the recipes and choose four or five soups that appeal to you, make them in advance, and freeze the extra portions for later use. If you freeze each portion separately, all you'll have to do is pop it in the microwave for a minute or two before your main course comes off the stove, and you'll have a hot starter that's as good as fresh.

Your Blender Is Your Friend

Many of us rarely use a blender except to make the occasional frozen cocktail, but on the Bikini Bootcamp meal plans you'll often find yourself using a blender once or twice a day. You will use it not only for your breakfast smoothies, but for salsas, dressings, soups, and the occasional dessert. So take your time and experiment with the different settings for different results. In general, you do not need to run the blender for more than a minute or two when blending salad dressings, though some vegetable soups may require three. If you like to retain some texture in your soups, do not blend them all the way—leave some of the veggies in small pieces rather than pureeing them entirely.

Preparing Fish or Chicken

The majority of our lunch and dinner recipes call for either grilled fish or chicken, and at Amansala we serve these at almost every meal. We're fans of grilling because when done properly (without extraordinarily high heat or charring), it greatly reduces the amount of fat in meat and makes lean protein even leaner. We recommend using an oven-top or a George Foreman grill if you have one; if that's not convenient, you can also steam, bake, or broil the fish or chicken using the broiler of your oven.

Any time you prepare fish or chicken, use the marinade of your choice from the Marinades section (see pages 261–63). All are tasty, versatile, and interchangeable with a variety of recipes, and the olive oil and citrus juices have additional health benefits. Believe it or not, using a citrus-based marinade actually reduces the formation of cancer-causing substances on meats and fish when they are cooked. If you're short on time, simply squeeze a little fresh lemon or lime juice over the meat or fish before you place it in the oven; when it comes out, sprinkle a little more juice on top and enjoy the natural flavors of your food.

Occasionally a recipe will call for boiled (or poached) chicken breasts, which is as easy as it sounds. Simply bring a pot of water to a boil, add the chicken, then decrease the heat and simmer for approximately seven minutes. Turn the chicken breasts over and simmer for approximately seven minutes on the other side or until cooked through. You can season the water with a few slices of fresh lemon if you wish; do not marinate the chicken before poaching.

Bikini Tip ....

When grilling, always brush olive oil over the surface of the grill before cooking to prevent the meat or fish from sticking.

....

Kitchen Time-Savers

- On Sunday, read the menus for the week ahead to familiarize your-self with what you will be making. Scan the pantry checklist on page 199, and head to the grocery store with your weekly shopping list.
- Do prep work ahead of time. You can prepare your soups and dress-ings in advance—say, in the morning before work or the night be-fore—so that they are ready to cook when it's time to eat.
- Some vegetables can be prepared ahead of time: Broccoli, cauli-flower, carrots, jicama, celery, and cucumber can all be cut up in ad-vance. Others, like tomatoes, avocados, ginger, and garlic, should be chopped only at the time of use. For those that can be prepped ahead of time, wash and store in Tupperware. Even if you don't worry about lunches and dinners, it's good to have carrot, jicama, or celery sticks on hand for emergency snacks.
- Lettuce and spinach can be washed in advance and stored in the fridge in sealable bags, where they will remain crisp for a day or two.
- Have your fruit washed and ready to eat. Papayas and pineapples can be cut into bite-size pieces in advance.
- If you plan to be out during the day, prepare your snacks in advance and take them with you in a sealable bag or Tupperware. If your workplace has a kitchen, stash your snacks in the refrigerator so you're never without something healthy to reach for when cravings kick in.

Now that you've reviewed our cooking basics, let's move on to the shopping lists. It's time to start assembling the ingredients to make your Bikini-friendly recipes a reality!

In Your Pantry

Before going shopping for your first week, you will need to clean out your kitchen cabinets and get rid of the old to make room for the new: new ingredients, new ways of eating, and new ways of looking at food. Any food that is not a part of your Bikini Bootcamp lifestyle must be tossed out—so open your fridge and your cupboards and start purging! Don't forget to eliminate any secret stashes of junk food, like candies in your desk drawer at work. Once you have removed all food that does not serve your greater purpose, you are ready to stock up on those that do.

The shopping lists that follow provide a rundown of specific, perish-able items you'll need for the weeks ahead. However, you may already have a few staples on your pantry shelves that you will want to have around no matter what. Before you head to the store for the first time, take note of which items you already have on hand to avoid doubling up on more costly foodstuffs, like olive oil or white wine.

Here are the basics you should have in your kitchen at all times:

Condiments:	Olive oil, extra virgin
	High-grade dark or toasted sesame oil
	Balsamic vinegar
	White wine vinegar
	Dry white wine or cooking wine
	Low-sodium soy sauce
	All-natural peanut butter (no added sugar)
	Brown sugar
	Honey
	Stevia or another sweetener
Spices:	Salt
	Freshly ground black pepper
	Oregano
	Curry powder
	Turmeric
	Cinnamon
Grains:	Whole-grain couscous
	Cereal, cold, 9 or 7-grain, high-fiber with at least 4 g. of fiber per serving, such as Kashi, 1 box
	Ak-Mak or other high-fiber, low-caloric crackers
Miscellaneous:	Green tea
	Hibiscus tea, or dried hibiscus flowers for brewing
	Aluminum foil
	Metal or wooden skewers for kebab recipes
	Nonstick cooking spray

When Shopping, Always Read the Labels

Be sure to check the labels on all packaged products to determine whether they contain any hidden sugars and to assess the fiber content. Ideally, any grains you buy should contain at least 4 grams of fiber per serving.

Week One Shopping List

Remember that our recipes are based on breakfast and lunch for one, dinner and dessert for two. So if you are going to be cooking dinner for more than two people, or lunch for more than one, you will need to go through and adjust the quantities. Also keep in mind that the list that follows assumes you are following the plan to the letter—a different soup every single day, a different dinner every day instead of eating leftovers, and so on. Use it as a starting point, but make adjustments to reflect your individual plan for the week ahead.

While most produce will keep for a week, you should be vigilant about the sell-by dates for all chicken and fish. You may want to buy your lean protein separately two or three times a week to avoid having it spoil.

Produce:
Apples, 2
Avocados, 5
Bananas, 3
Blueberries, 1 pt.
Broccoli, 2 large heads
Carrots, full-sized, 4 lbs. or 4 bags (2 lbs. or
    2 bags if not making Carrot Ginger Soup)
Cauliflower, 1 large head
Celery, 1 bunch
Cilantro, fresh, 2 bunches
Cucumber, 1
Garlic, 2 heads
Ginger root, 2 large
Jalapeño or serrano green chili peppers,
    6 (optional)

Jicamas, 2

Lemons, 3

Lettuce, romaine, 2 heads

Limes, 7

Mangoes, 2

Mint, fresh, 1 small bunch

Mushrooms, white button, medium, 1 lb. or
2 containers

Napa cabbage, 2

Onions, medium, 5

Onions, large, 2

Oranges, 2

Papaya, 1

Pepper, green bell, 1

Pepper, red bell, 1

Pineapple, 1

Raisins, 1/2 lb.

Spinach, fresh, 5 bunches

Tomatoes, 20 (less if not making White Bean
& Roasted Tomato Soup or all salsas)

Tomatoes, cherry, 1 pt.

Tomatoes, plum, 2 (if making Sopa de Lima)

Watermelon, 1/4

Zucchini, medium, 1

Zucchini, large, 1

Bikini Tip

Since many of our recipes call for garlic, you can save time by buying pre-minced garlic in a jar (packed in water). Some grocery stores also sell minced, prepped ginger—another key ingredient in many Bikini meals.

Nuts, Seeds, & Grains:	Almonds, crushed or sliced, 1/2 lb.
	Almonds, whole, 1/2 lb.
	Amaranth cooked cereal (found in health food stores. If unavailable, substitute a 9-grain, high-fiber breakfast cereal such as Kashi.)
	Flax seeds, 1/2 lb.
	Pumpkin seeds, toasted, 1/2 lb.
	Sesame seeds, toasted, 1/2 lb.
	Soba noodles, one 12-oz. pkg.
Beans:	Black beans, three 15-oz. cans or one 16-oz. pkg. dried
	Chickpeas (garbanzo beans), two 15-oz. cans
	Lentils, dried, one 16-oz. pkg.
	White beans, two 15-oz. cans
Meat & Fish:	Chicken breasts, 5–6 oz., skinless boneless, 7
	Fish fillets, white, 5–6 oz., 8
	Shrimp, 10, large
	Tuna, packed in water, one 6-oz. can
	Eggs, 1 doz.
Dairy:	Yogurt, low-fat plain or vanilla, one 32-oz. container (we like Total Greek Yogurt with 2% fat)
	Milk, nonfat, 1/2 gallon
Miscellaneous:	Caramel sauce, one 12-oz. jar
	Chicken broth, low-sodium, four 32-oz. cartons
For Spa Treats:	Avocado, 1
	Cucumber, 1
	Kiwi, 1
	Papaya, 1
	An essential oil such as lavender or chamomile, *or* chamomile tea bags
	Unscented body lotion
	Scented candles

When buying pumpkin seeds, make sure they were not roasted in oil or honey. If in doubt, ask.

Week Two Shopping List

Take an inventory of your fridge to get ready for Week Two. Read through the menus and check to see if you have any vegetables left over from Week One that are still fresh. Ginger root stays fresh for weeks if refrigerated, and so do garlic, cabbage, lemons, and limes. Remember that this list assumes you are making the full menu top to bottom every day, with a new soup for each day and no leftovers from prior meals. So review it carefully and adjust the quantities

Produce:
Apples, 2
Avocados, 5
Bananas, 2
Blueberries, frozen, 12-oz. bag
Broccoli, 1 large head
Carrots, full-size, two 1-lb. bags
Cauliflower, 1 large head
Celery, 1 bunch
Cilantro, fresh, 2 bunches
Cucumbers, 5
Garlic, 2 heads
Ginger root, 2 large
Jalapeño or serrano green chili peppers,
    9 (optional)
Jicamas, 2
Lemons, 3
Lettuce, romaine, 2 heads
Limes, 14
Mangoes, 4

Mint, fresh, 1 bunch

Mushrooms, 6 white button, medium

Napa cabbage, 2 heads

Onions, medium, 6

Onions, large, 3

Orange, 1

Pear, 1

Pepper, green bell, 3

Pepper, yellow bell, 1

Pineapple, 1

Radishes, large red, 6

Raisins, 1/2 lb.

Scallions, 1 bunch

Spinach, 3 bunches

Squash, butternut, 1 medium

Tomatoes, medium, 16

Tomatoes, large, 7

Tomatoes, diced, two 14-oz. cans

Watermelon, 1/4

Zucchini, medium, 2

Zucchini, large, 5

Nuts, Seeds & Grains: Peanuts, crushed, 1/4 lb.

Soba noodles, one 12-oz. pkg.

Tortillas, stone-ground (corn, not
flour-based), 6

Walnuts, chopped, 1/4 lb.

Beans: Black beans, five 15-oz. cans

Chickpeas (garbanzo beans), three 15-oz. cans

Meat & Fish: Chicken breasts, 5–6 oz., skinless, boneless, 10

Fish fillets, white, 5–6 oz., 7

Dairy: Milk, nonfat, 1 qt. (if last week's milk has
expired)

	Yogurt, low-fat plain or vanilla, one 32 oz. container (we like Total Greek Yogurt with 2% fat)
Miscellaneous:	Chicken broth, low-sodium, three 32-oz. containers
	Coconut, shredded, no added sugar (can also buy a fresh coconut and grate)
For Spa Treats:	Carrot, 1 large
	Tomato, 1
	Oatmeal, dried
	Granulated sugar, small pkg.
	Jasmine flowers, dried (available at Asian or health food stores)
	Sweet almond oil
	Jasmine essential oil
	Rose petals, dried
	Purifying clay mask (any brand)
	A dry body brush, available in health food stores

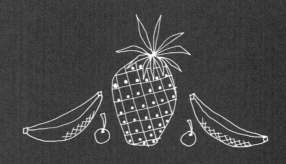

Breakfasts

AMARANTH COOKED CEREAL
Makes 1 serving

Amaranth-based cereals, which cook like oatmeal or cream of wheat, can be found at many supermarkets and health food stores. Cooking instructions vary, so be sure to check the package on your particular brand.

1 cup amaranth cereal
1 cup water or 1/2 cup skim milk and 1/2 cup water

Cook according to the package instructions.

BANANA SMOOTHIE
Makes 1 serving

A fruit smoothie is a great all-in-one breakfast or anytime treat that satisfies cravings for sweets and delivers plenty of nutrition. You can use this recipe to experiment with other fruits to create your personal favorite. At Bikini Bootcamp, we love to experiment with native fruits, such as papaya, pineapple, and mango. Flax seeds provide additional fiber, which leaves you feeling sated, and also deliver a dose of healthy omega-3s.

1 banana
1/2 cup low-fat milk, soy milk, or low-fat plain or vanilla yogurt
1 cup crushed ice
Dollop of honey, if needed
1 teaspoon flax seeds

1. Place all the ingredients in a blender and blend on high until smooth.
2. Pour into a tall glass and serve.

BANANA SWIRL
Makes 1 serving

This tasty treat—flavored with cinnamon to appease your sweet tooth—makes a filling breakfast.

1/2 cup low-fat plain or vanilla yogurt

1 banana, sliced

1 tablespoon cinnamon

1 tablespoon low-fat, high-fiber cold cereal

1. Spoon the yogurt over the banana slices and sprinkle with the cinnamon and cereal.
2. Mix together and serve.

BANANA YOGURT PARFAIT
Makes 1 serving

Believe it or not, bananas and ginger go wonderfully together, and the almonds and amaranth give this breakfast a satisfying crunch.

1 banana, sliced

1/2 cup low-fat plain or vanilla yogurt

1 teaspoon freshly grated ginger

1 teaspoon sliced almonds

1 tablespoon high-fiber, 9-grain cold cereal

1. Combine the banana, yogurt, and ginger in a blender and blend until smooth. Transfer to a bowl.
2. Serve sprinkled with the almonds and cereal.

BLUEBERRY SMOOTHIE
Makes 1 serving

Blueberry smoothies give you a healthy dose of one of nature's "super foods" to start your day. Don't forget to add some extra fiber, such as flax seeds, to ensure that you feel satisfied.

1 cup fresh or frozen (with no added sugar) blueberries
1/2 cup low-fat milk or low-fat plain or vanilla yogurt
1 cup crushed ice
Dollop of honey, if needed
1 teaspoon flax seeds

1. Place all the ingredients in a blender and blend on high until smooth.
2. Pour into a tall glass and serve.

FRUIT BOWL WITH ALMONDS
Makes 1 serving

Select from the season's freshest fruits, or use any leftovers you may have, and savor their tastes as you start your day.

1 cup combination any fresh fruit: sliced bananas, blueberries, pineapple chunks, mango chunks, sliced apple, sliced papaya
1 tablespoon sliced almonds

1. Combine the fruit in a bowl and toss well.
2. Sprinkle with the almonds and serve.

GINGER PINEAPPLE SMOOTHIE

Makes 1 serving

The ginger in this smoothie cleanses the blood and gives you a nice kick with which to start the day.

1/4 cup pineapple chunks
1 teaspoon chopped ginger
1/2 cup low-fat plain or vanilla yogurt
1 tablespoon flax seeds

1. Combine all the ingredients in a blender and blend until smooth.
2. Pour into a glass and serve.

HARD-BOILED EGGS WITH SALSA MEXICANA

Makes 1 serving

This variation on traditional egg salad is simple and full of protein. Make the eggs ahead of time and keep them in the fridge if you are pressed for time in the mornings.

2 hard-boiled eggs, peeled
Salsa Mexicana (see page 267)

1. Chop the eggs into bite-size pieces.
2. Spoon salsa over the eggs and serve.

HUEVOS MEXICANA

Makes 1 serving

What would Bikini Bootcamp be without this tasty Mexican specialty? If you're not a fan of spicy foods for breakfast, simply leave out the jalapeño. This is also great for a weekend treat when you have a little more time to savor breakfast.

1 tablespoon extra virgin olive oil
1/4 cup chopped onion
1 tablespoon minced jalapeño pepper
2 eggs
Salt and freshly ground black pepper
1/4 cup chopped tomatoes
Small handful fresh cilantro leaves

1. Heat the oil in a large skillet over medium heat. Add the onion and jalapeño and sauté, stirring frequently, for 2 to 3 minutes, until the vegetables are soft but not browned. Decrease the heat to medium-low.
2. Whisk together the eggs, salt, and pepper in a bowl.
3. Add the eggs to the skillet and stir for 4 to 5 minutes, or until the eggs are almost set. Add the tomatoes and cilantro. Stir again and cook for 2 more minutes, or until the eggs are set. Serve immediately.

MANGO MADNESS SMOOTHIE
Makes 1 serving

Here's a Mexican-style smoothie. If you can't get enough mango, this one's for you.

1 cup chopped mango
1/2 cup low-fat milk
1 cup crushed ice
Sweetener, if needed

1. Place all the ingredients in a blender and blend on high until smooth.
2. Pour into a glass and serve.

MANGO YOGURT PARFAIT
Makes 1 serving

This low-cal but delicious breakfast gives you 4 grams of fiber!

1/2 cup low-fat plain or vanilla yogurt
1 cup diced mango
2 tablespoons high-fiber cold cereal

Spoon the yogurt over the mango, sprinkle with the cereal, and serve.

PINEAPPLE SWIRL
Makes 1 serving

This tropical delight will jump-start your day.

1/2 cup low-fat plain or vanilla yogurt
1 cup pineapple chunks
1 tablespoon low-fat, high-fiber cold cereal

1. Spoon the yogurt over the pineapple and sprinkle with cereal.
2. Mix together and serve.

SCRAMBLED EGGS WITH SPINACH & MUSHROOMS
Makes 1 serving

Start your day with protein! If you have your spinach and mushrooms washed and ready in the fridge, this delicious breakfast takes no more than 5 minutes to prepare.

1 tablespoon extra virgin olive oil

4 to 5 white button mushrooms, washed, patted dry, and sliced

2 eggs

Salt and freshly ground black pepper

Small handful fresh spinach leaves, washed and chopped

1 cup chopped tomatoes (optional)

1. Heat the oil in a large skillet over medium-high heat. Add the mushrooms and sauté, stirring frequently, for 2 to 3 minutes, until the mushrooms are soft. Decrease the heat to medium.
2. Whisk together the eggs, salt, and pepper in a medium bowl.
3. Add the eggs to the skillet and stir for 4 to 5 minutes, or until the eggs are almost set. Add the spinach and tomatoes, if desired. Stir again and cook for 2 more minutes, or until the eggs are set. Serve immediately.

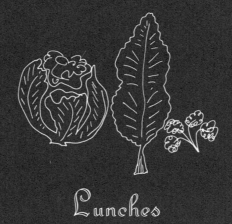

Lunches

AMANSALA SALAD WITH GINGER-SESAME DRESSING

Makes 1 serving

This fabulous salad is the most requested recipe in our Bikini Bootcamp repertoire! It works great with either grilled fish or chicken, and over the course of the program, you'll enjoy it both ways. It packs quality nutrition into very few calories, plus it delivers a hefty dose of healthy fiber to fill you up so you're never hungry. We guarantee that you'll be making it long after these two weeks are up!

1 cup shredded Napa cabbage

1 cup shredded romaine lettuce

1/2 cup shredded carrots

1/2 cup diced tomatoes

1/4 cup diced avocado (optional)

1 5- to 6-ounce piece grilled fish or chicken, chopped (page 197)

Ginger-Sesame Dressing (page 259)

1 tablespoon toasted sesame seeds

1. Combine the cabbage, lettuce, carrots, tomatoes, avocado, and fish or chicken in a large bowl and toss with the dressing to taste.
2. Sprinkle with the toasted sesame seeds and serve.

ASIAN CHICKEN LETTUCE WRAPS WITH CRUSHED PEANUTS

Makes 1 serving

These high-protein wraps are fun to eat and filling.

1 tablespoon extra virgin olive oil

1 teaspoon toasted sesame oil

1 garlic clove, minced

1 teaspoon minced ginger

1 stalk celery, finely chopped

1/2 cup shredded carrot

5 to 6 ounces ground chicken (if unavailable, chop a 5- to 6-ounce boneless breast into the smallest pieces you can)

Salt and freshly ground black pepper

3 large leaves romaine lettuce, washed and dried (best if washed and stored in the fridge ahead of time)

2 tablespoons peanuts, crushed

1. Heat the olive and sesame oils in a large skillet over medium heat. Add the garlic and ginger and sauté for 5 minutes, stirring frequently.
2. Add the celery, carrot, and chicken and cook for 5 minutes, or until the chicken is cooked through. Season with salt and pepper to taste.
3. Remove from heat and divide the chicken mixture among the three lettuce leaves. Spoon the mixture onto the center of each leaf, sprinkle with crushed peanuts, and then roll burrito-style, or fold over like a taco. Serve immediately.

BLACK BEAN SALAD
Makes 1 serving

Rich in fiber, black beans keep your blood sugar stable, which means you feel full longer, and they are the richest in antioxidants of all beans. This tasty salad is simple to prepare; make it a couple of hours or the night before and let the flavors mingle.

DRESSING

2 tablespoons fresh lemon juice

1 tablespoon extra virgin olive oil

1 tablespoon toasted pumpkin seeds, chopped

Small handful fresh cilantro leaves, chopped

SALAD

1/2 (15-ounce) can black beans, drained and rinsed

1 tomato, chopped

1/2 cup finely chopped onion

1/2 cup diced red bell pepper

1 garlic clove, minced

Salt and freshly ground black pepper

1. To make the dressing, whisk together all the dressing ingredients in a bowl. Set aside.
2. To make the salad, combine the black beans, tomato, onion, bell pepper, and garlic in a bowl. Mix and toss with dressing.
3. Season to taste with salt and pepper and serve.

CHICKEN TACO SALAD

Makes 1 serving

Tastes so good and fresh you won't even miss the taco shell! If you're not a fan of salsa, top with a squeeze of fresh lime juice instead.

1 cup shredded or finely chopped Napa cabbage

1/2 cup shredded romaine lettuce

1/2 (15-ounce) can black beans, drained and rinsed

1 tomato, cubed

1/4 avocado, cubed

1 5- to 6-ounce chicken breast, boiled and shredded (page 197)

1 tablespoon extra virgin olive oil

Salt and freshly ground black pepper

Salsa Mexicana (page 267)

1. Combine the cabbage, lettuce, beans, tomato, avocado, and chicken in a bowl. Toss with the oil and season to taste with salt and pepper.
2. Add salsa to taste and serve.

CHOPPED VEGETABLE & CHICKPEA SALAD WITH CITRUS DRESSING
Makes 1 serving

The citrus dressing blends nicely with the nutty flavor of the chickpeas. Light and fresh, this salad makes a great warm-weather treat.

1/2 (15-ounce) can chickpeas (garbanzo beans), drained and rinsed

1/4 jicama, peeled and cut into 1/4-inch cubes (or substitute celery)

1/2 cucumber, peeled, seeded, and cut into 1/4-inch cubes

1 medium tomato, chopped

1/2 cup minced cilantro leaves (optional)

Citrus Dressing (page 258)

Salt and freshly ground black pepper

1. Combine the chickpeas, jicama, cucumber, tomato, and cilantro in a large bowl. Toss with the dressing to taste.
2. Season with salt and pepper and serve immediately.

COUSCOUS SALAD WITH MINT, RAISINS, & ALMONDS
Makes 1 serving

Couscous is filling and a great source of fat-free fiber. The mint in this Moroccan-style dish gives it a nice fresh taste.

1/2 cup whole-grain couscous

1/2 cup raisins

1/2 (15-ounce) can chickpeas (garbanzo beans), drained and rinsed

1/2 cucumber, cubed

1/4 cup (small handful) fresh mint, finely chopped

1 tablespoon sliced almonds

Curry Dressing (page 258)

1. Prepare the couscous according to the instructions on box.
2. Soak the raisins in warm water to cover for 10 minutes to soften, then drain.
3. Mix together the couscous, raisins, chickpeas, cucumber, mint, almonds, and dressing to taste in a large bowl. Toss lightly with a large fork so the couscous isn't broken up too much. Serve at room temperature.

CRUNCHY CHICKEN SALAD WITH RAISINS & APPLES
Makes 1 serving

The apples and pumpkin seeds provide a satisfying crunch in this simple Middle Eastern style salad. For variety, substitute jicama for the apple.

1/3 cup raisins

1 5- to 6-ounce chicken breast, boiled and shredded (p. 197)

1 small apple, peeled, cored, and cubed

1 stalk celery, diced

2 tablespoons toasted pumpkin seeds

Curry Dressing (page 258)

1. Soak the raisins in warm water to cover for 10 minutes to soften, then drain.
2. Combine the raisins, chicken, apple, celery, and pumpkin seeds in a large bowl and toss with the dressing to taste.
3. Serve immediately or store in the refrigerator for several days.

CURRIED SPINACH SALAD WITH PAPAYA & PUMPKIN SEEDS
Makes 1 serving

This easy-to-make salad delivers plenty of iron and other vitamins we women need, especially when we're engaged in an intensive shape-up plan. Top with either grilled fish or chicken.

1 (5-ounce) bag baby spinach or regular fresh spinach, tough stems discarded, washed and dried
1 papaya, peeled, pitted, and cubed (or substitute another fruit, such as mango or pear)
1/4 cup toasted pumpkin seeds
1 5- to 6-ounce grilled white fish fillet or chicken breast (page 197)
Curry Dressing (page 258)

1. Combine the spinach, papaya, pumpkin seeds, and fish or chicken in a large bowl.
2. Toss with the dressing to taste. Serve immediately.

Bikini Tip

When preparing this dish with chicken, shred the chicken into bite-size pieces and toss with all the ingredients to allow the heat of the chicken to wilt the spinach. This makes a great "warm" salad.

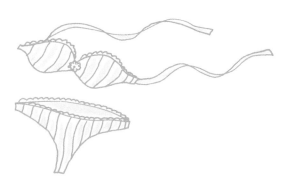

FRESH SPINACH & CHICKPEA SALAD WITH TOMATOES & WALNUTS

Makes 1 serving

This refreshing salad tastes best with walnuts, but pumpkin seeds add a nice crunch as well.

1 cup fresh packed spinach leaves, washed and dried

1/2 (15-ounce) can chickpeas, drained and rinsed

1 medium tomato, chopped

1 tablespoon raisins

1 tablespoon chopped walnuts or toasted pumpkin seeds

Orange-Cilantro Dressing (page 260)

1. Combine the spinach, chickpeas, tomato, raisins, and walnuts in a large bowl.
2. Toss with the dressing to taste and serve.

JICAMA, BLACK BEAN, & AVOCADO SALAD

Makes 1 serving

With the smooth avocado and the crunchy jicama, this delicious, simple salad is rich in texture and takes just minutes to prepare.

1/4 jicama, peeled and cubed

1 medium tomato, chopped

1/2 (15-ounce) can black beans, drained and rinsed

1/2 avocado, cubed

Orange-Cilantro Dressing (page 260)

Salt and freshly ground black pepper

1. Combine the jicama, tomato, black beans, and avocado in a large bowl.
2. Toss with the dressing to taste. Add salt and pepper to taste, and serve.

MANGO CHICKEN SALAD

Makes 1 serving

Mangoes provide a bit of sweetness for this salad. If mangoes are not readily available in your area, oranges will do the trick as well.

2 cups shredded romaine lettuce

1/2 mango, cubed (or substitute another fruit if mango is not available)

1 tablespoon sliced almonds

1 5- to 6-ounce grilled chicken breast, shredded (page 197)

Mango-Orange Dressing (page 259)

1. Combine the lettuce, mango, almonds, and chicken in a large bowl.
2. Toss with the dressing to taste and serve immediately.

SOBA NOODLE SALAD WITH SESAME CHICKEN

Makes 1 serving

Japanese buckwheat noodles, called soba, are found in health-food stores and the Asian section of most grocery stores. They are wheat-free, so they are a great alternative for anyone who is allergic to wheat or gluten. Take note: They cook quickly and must be watched.

1/4 (12-ounce) package soba noodles

3 to 4 broccoli florets, cut into bite-size pieces

1 5- to 6-ounce chicken breast, boiled and shredded (p. 197)

1 cup shredded or finely chopped Napa cabbage

1 carrot, shredded

Ginger-Sesame Dressing (page 259)

1 tablespoon toasted sesame seeds

1. Bring a large pot of water to a boil and add the soba noodles. Cook until tender, about 3 minutes. Do not overcook as soba cooks faster than Italian pasta. Drain immediately and run under cool water.
2. In separate small pan, drop broccoli in enough water to cover and bring to a boil. Boil for 3 minutes, or just enough to retain its green color and soften slightly. Drain and run under cold water until cool.
3. If the soba noodles become sticky, run hot water over them to loosen. Combine the noodles, chicken, broccoli, cabbage, and carrot in a large bowl.
4. Toss the salad with the dressing until coated. Sprinkle with sesame seeds and serve.

WHITE BEAN & TUNA SALAD IN ORANGE-CILANTRO DRESSING
Makes 1 serving

This easy-to-make salad packs in the protein and tastes delicious.

1/2 (15-ounce) can cannellini beans, drained and rinsed
1 (6-ounce) can tuna packed in water, drained
1 carrot, shredded
1/2 cucumber, peeled, seeded, and cubed
2 tablespoons diced jicama
Orange-Cilantro Dressing (page 260)

Toss all the ingredients together in a large bowl with dressing to taste and serve immediately.

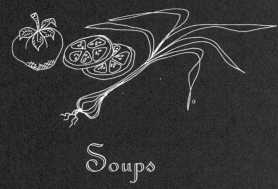

Soups

BLACK BEAN SOUP

Makes 4 servings

This classic Mexican soup is made with fiber-rich black beans. While you can use dried beans, which require advance cooking as well as presoaking overnight (see recipe on page 265), this easy version uses canned beans. The results are equally flavorful.

1 tablespoon extra virgin olive oil

1/4 large onion, chopped

1 teaspoon diced green chile (optional)

2 garlic cloves, chopped

2 (15-ounce) cans black beans, drained and rinsed

3 cups low-sodium chicken broth

Salt and freshly ground black pepper

1 avocado, diced

1/2 jicama, diced

1 medium tomato, diced

2 tablespoons minced fresh cilantro

1. Heat the oil in a large saucepan over medium heat. Add the onion, chile, if using, and garlic and sauté for 5 to 7 minutes, until the onion is translucent and not burned.
2. Add the beans, and the broth, decrease the heat to low, and cook for 10 minutes.
3. Remove from the heat and let cool for 10 minutes.
4. Working in batches, transfer the soup to a food processor or blender and process until smooth.
5. Return the puree to the saucepan and heat for 5 minutes over medium heat. If necessary, thin with water. Season with salt and pepper.
6. Garnish each serving with avocado, jicama, tomato, and cilantro, if you like.

Blending Soups

When blending soup in a food processor or blender, follow these steps:

1. Remove the soup from the heat and transfer into a large bowl or similarly sized pan or pot. Allow the soup to cool for 10 minutes.

2. Working in batches, transfer the soup to a blender and blend for 1 to 2 minutes. You want to be sure to only half fill the blender each time and use a lid so the liquid does not splash out and burn you. Each time you blend, start on slow and increase to a higher speed.

3. Return the blended soup to the original saucepan and move on to the next batch.

Note: If you like more texture to your soups, you can blend for less time. If you need to thin the soup, add a little more broth or water.

BROCCOLI SOUP

Makes 4 servings

While broccoli is the cornerstone of this tasty recipe, you get additional fiber, flavor, and color from the cabbage and cauliflower..

1 medium to large head broccoli, broken into florets

1/2 small head cauliflower, broken into florets

1/4 head Napa cabbage, coarsely chopped or broken

1/4 onion, chopped

1 garlic clove, minced

3 cups low-sodium chicken broth

Salt and freshly ground black pepper

Toasted sesame seeds or pumpkin seeds, for garnish

1. In a large saucepan, combine the broccoli, cauliflower, cabbage, onion, and garlic. Add the broth, either the 3 cups or enough to cover the vegetables.

2. Bring to a boil, then decrease the heat to medium and cook, uncovered, for 20 to 25 minutes, until the vegetables are tender. Remove the soup from the heat and let cool for 10 minutes.

3. Working in batches, transfer the soup to a food processor or blender and process until smooth.

4. Return the soup to the saucepan. Cook over medium heat for 5 minutes longer. Season with salt and pepper.
5. Top each serving with a sprinkle of toasted sesame seeds or pumpkin seeds. Serve immediately.

BUTTERNUT SQUASH SOUP
Makes 4 servings

Traditionally a cold-weather favorite, this tasty soup is enjoyed on our sunny shores as well.

1 tablespoon extra virgin olive oil

1/2 large onion, chopped

1 garlic clove, minced

1 thumb-sized piece ginger, peeled and minced

2 tablespoons brown sugar

1 medium butternut squash, peeled and cut into chunks

3 cups low-sodium chicken broth

Salt and freshly ground black pepper to taste

Toasted pumpkin seeds, for garnish

1. Heat the oil in a large saucepan over medium heat. Add the onion, garlic, and ginger, and sauté, stirring frequently, for 6 to 8 minutes, until the onion is soft but not browned. Stir in the brown sugar. Set aside.
2. Cook the squash in a large pot with the broth until tender, 25 to 30 minutes.
3. Remove the squash from the heat, but do not drain. Let cool for 10 minutes. Add the garlic-ginger mixture.
4. Working in batches, transfer the soup to a food processor or a blender and process until smooth.
5. Return the soup to the pot and cook over medium heat for 5 minutes longer. Season with salt and pepper.
6. Top each serving with a sprinkle of toasted pumpkin seeds. Serve immediately.

CARROT GINGER SOUP

Makes 4 servings

Noted for its unique flavor and antioxidant properties, the ginger in this recipe meshes well with the sweetness of the carrots.

4 large, thick carrots, sliced

3 cups low-sodium chicken broth

1 tablespoon extra virgin olive oil

1/2 large onion, chopped

2 garlic cloves, minced

2 tablespoons peeled, minced ginger

2 tablespoons brown sugar

Salt and freshly ground black pepper to taste

Toasted pumpkin seeds, for garnish

1. Cook the carrots in a large pot with the broth until tender, 25 to 30 minutes.
2. Remove from the heat and let cool for 10 minutes.
3. While the carrots cook, heat the oil in a large saucepan over medium heat. Add the onion, garlic, and 1 tablespoon of the ginger, and sauté, stirring frequently, for 6 to 8 minutes, until the onion is soft but not browned.
4. Working in batches, transfer the carrots and the cooked garlic-ginger mixture and the remaining 1 tablespoon of uncooked ginger to a food processor or blender. Blend for 2 to 3 minutes until smooth.
5. Return the soup to the saucepan and add the brown sugar. Stir until the sugar dissolves and cook for 5 minutes over medium heat. Season with salt and pepper.
6. Top each serving with a sprinkle of toasted pumpkin seeds. Serve immediately.

CAULIFLOWER SOUP
Makes 4 servings

The nutty, rich flavor of the cauliflower makes this soup a satisfying beginning to any meal.

1/2 large head cauliflower, cut into florets

1/4 head Napa cabbage, shredded

1/4 onion

1 celery stalk, finely chopped

1 tablespoon minced garlic

3 cups low-sodium chicken broth

1 teaspoon curry powder (optional)

Salt and freshly ground black pepper

Toasted pumpkin or sesame seeds, for garnish

1. In a large saucepan, combine the cauliflower, cabbage, onion, celery, and garlic. Add the chicken broth, either 3 cups or enough to cover.
2. Bring to a boil, then decrease the heat to medium and cook, uncovered, for 20 to 25 minutes, until the vegetables are tender. Remove from the heat and let cool for 10 minutes.
3. Working in batches, transfer the soup to a food processor or blender and process until smooth.
4. Return the soup to the saucepan. Add the curry powder, if using. Cook for 5 minutes longer. Season with salt and pepper.
5. Top each serving with a sprinkle of toasted pumpkin seeds. Serve immediately.

CLEAR CHICKEN SOUP WITH LIME & AVOCADO
Makes 4 servings

This simple chicken soup makes good use of traditional Mexican toppings.

3 cups low-sodium chicken broth

1 small serrano or jalapeño chile, seeded and minced

Salt and freshly ground black pepper

1/2 avocado, diced

2 tablespoons chopped fresh cilantro leaves

2 tablespoons chopped tomato

1 lime, quartered

1. Heat the chicken broth over medium-high heat. Add the chile and bring to a boil. Decrease the heat to medium and simmer for about 15 minutes.
2. Season with salt and pepper as needed.
3. Ladle the broth into bowls and top with the avocado, cilantro, tomato, and a squeeze of lime.

GAZPACHO
Makes 4 servings

This light, healthy soup is refreshing any time of the year. We recommend making it a few hours ahead so the flavors can mingle. Serve it chilled. It also makes a great snack!

6 large tomatoes, chopped

1 medium yellow bell pepper, diced

1 cucumber, peeled, seeded, and diced

1/2 medium onion, finely minced

1 jalapeño, seeded and chopped (optional)

2 medium garlic cloves, pressed

2 tablespoons chopped fresh cilantro leaves

1/4 cup fresh lemon juice

1 tablespoon extra virgin olive oil

1/4 jicama, peeled and diced for topping

4 tablespoons low-fat plain yogurt (optional)

1. Combine the tomatoes, bell pepper, cucumber, onion, jalapeño, if using, garlic, cilantro, lemon juice, and oil in a large bowl.
2. Transfer half of the mixture to a blender or food processor and blend for 1 minute; then return to bowl and mix well.
3. Top each portion with the jicama and yogurt before serving.

Bikini Tip

At Amansala, we blend only half the mixture so the soup retains a chunky texture. If you prefer a smoother gazpacho, simply blend the entire batch.

LENTIL SOUP

Makes 4 servings

To add some additional flavor to this already yummy soup, or for a little variety, substitute low-sodium chicken broth for water, or add 1 teaspoon curry powder.

1 zucchini, diced

1 carrot, diced

1/2 onion, diced

1 cup dried lentils

Salt and freshly ground black pepper

1. Place the vegetables and lentils in a soup pot and cover with 4 cups water.
2. Bring to a boil, then decrease the heat to simmer for 1 hour, or until the lentils become tender. If the lentils become too thick, add more water to the consistency that you like.
3. Season with salt and pepper. Serve hot.

MUSHROOM SPINACH SOUP
Makes 4 servings

The cauliflower adds nice body to this iron-packed, delicious soup.

3 cups low-sodium chicken broth

1/2 cup chopped cauliflower florets

1/2 cup chopped broccoli florets

1/2 onion, diced

1 teaspoon peeled, minced ginger

2 teaspoons minced garlic

1 tablespoon extra virgin olive oil

10 white button mushrooms, cut into bite-sized pieces

2 cups packed, chopped fresh spinach

Salt and freshly ground black pepper

Toasted pumpkin seeds, for garnish

1. Bring the chicken broth to a boil in a large saucepan and add the cauliflower, broccoli, onion, ginger, and 1 teaspoon of the garlic. Cook over medium heat for 20 minutes.
2. Meanwhile, in a small saucepan over medium heat, heat the oil. Add the remaining 1 teaspoon garlic and sauté for about 1 minute. Add the mushrooms and sauté for about 3 minutes, or until they are soft. Turn off the heat and stir in the spinach.
3. Remove the chicken broth mixture from the heat and allow to cool for 10 minutes. Working in batches, transfer the broth and vegetable mixture to a blender or food processor, and blend until smooth.

4. Return the broth mixture to the pot, and cook for 5 minutes over medium heat. Stir the spinach and mushrooms into the hot soup. Season with salt and pepper.
5. Top each serving with a sprinkle of toasted pumpkin seeds.

SOPA DE LIMA
Makes 4 servings

This refreshing soup gets its zing from the fresh lime cooked into it, peel and all. Keep the soup focused on the veggies if you want to keep things light; or add the chicken for a heartier meal.

1 tablespoon extra virgin olive oil

1/2 large onion, chopped

1/2 green bell pepper, cut into 1-inch pieces

1/2 large zucchini, cut into 1-inch pieces

2 large plum tomatoes, cut into 1-inch pieces

1 celery stalk, chopped

2 garlic cloves, minced

Freshly ground black pepper

1 32-ounce box low-sodium chicken broth

6 limes

2 5- to 6-ounce boneless, skinless chicken breast halves (optional)

Salt

1. In a large saucepan over medium heat, warm the oil. Add the onion, bell pepper, zucchini, tomatoes, celery, and garlic. Season with pepper, and sauté, stirring frequently to coat, for 4 to 5 minutes, until tender.
2. Add enough broth to cover the vegetables. Slice 4 of the limes into four rounds each and add to the soup. Add the chicken breasts, if using, and bring to a boil. Decrease the heat to medium and cook, covered, for 25 to 30 minutes, or until the chicken is cooked through.

3. Remove the chicken breasts and let cool.
4. Juice the remaining 2 limes and remove any seeds. Add the lime juice to the soup and season with salt. Cook for 5 minutes. Remove the lime slices.
5. Shred the cooled chicken into bite-size pieces. To serve, place a slice of lime and the shredded chicken at the bottom of four shallow bowls and ladle in the soup. Serve immediately.

SPICY MEXICAN VEGETABLE SOUP
Makes 4 servings

The chiles kick this recipe up a notch from traditional vegetable soup.

3 cups low-sodium chicken broth

1/2 onion, finely chopped

1/2 green bell pepper, diced

2 garlic cloves, chopped

1/2 zucchini, chopped

2 (14-ounce) cans diced tomatoes in juice

2 jalapeño chiles, seeded and finely chopped (optional)

1 teaspoon dried oregano

Salt and freshly ground black pepper

2 tablespoons toasted pumpkin seeds

Large handful chopped fresh cilantro leaves

1 lime, quartered

1. In a large soup pot, combine 1/4 cup of the chicken broth with the onion, bell pepper, and garlic, and sauté over medium heat for about 7 minutes, or until the onion starts to wilt.
2. Add the zucchini, tomatoes, jalapeños, if using, oregano, and remaining chicken broth, and bring to a boil. Decrease the heat and simmer for 30 minutes.
3. Add salt and pepper to taste.
4. Serve hot with pumpkin seeds sprinkled on top, along with a sprinkle of cilantro and a squeeze of fresh lime.

TORTILLA-LESS TORTILLA SOUP
Makes 4 servings

Our Bikini Bootcamp campers love this vegetable soup—and so will you. It gets its rich, distinctive flavor from charring the vegetables before adding them to the soup.

6 large tomatoes, chopped

1/2 large onion, chopped

1 celery stalk, chopped

1 large carrot, chopped

Sea salt and freshly ground black pepper

1 tablespoon minced garlic

1/2 jicama, peeled and diced

1/2 avocado, cubed

1. Heat a large dry skillet over medium heat. Working in batches, char the tomatoes, onion, celery, and carrot for 8 to 10 minutes, until the tomatoes start to break open a bit and the onion looks a little charred. Season with salt and pepper. (A variation on this is to char the vegetables over a gas flame or place them on a hot grill.)
2. Transfer the mixture to a pot and add enough water to cover the vegetables. Add the garlic and cook over medium-high heat until the tomatoes have broken down, 20 to 25 minutes.
3. Remove the soup from the heat and let cool for 10 minutes. Working in batches, transfer the soup to a blender or food processor and puree on low for 15 seconds. Return the blended soup to the soup pot and cook for 5 more minutes. Season with salt and pepper.
4. Top each serving with the jicama and avocado. Serve immediately.

Note

To make this soup more of a meal, add one stone-ground corn tortilla, cut into strips, per person.

WHITE BEAN & ROASTED TOMATO SOUP
Makes 4 servings

The flavor of the roasted tomatoes makes this soup a stand-out dish.

4 to 6 medium tomatoes, cut in half lengthwise

1 large carrot, chopped

2 tablespoons extra virgin olive oil

1 tablespoon minced garlic

1/2 onion, chopped

1 stalk celery, chopped

3 cups low-sodium chicken broth

1 15-ounce can cannellini beans, drained and rinsed

Salt and freshly ground black pepper

1. Preheat the oven to 350° F.
2. In a medium bowl, combine the tomatoes, carrot, 1 tablespoon of the oil, and 1 teaspoon of the garlic and mix to coat.
3. Place the tomato and carrot mixture in a roasting pan and roast for about 45 minutes, or until the tomatoes are almost blackened and very soft.
4. When the tomatoes and carrots are close to being done, heat the remaining 1 tablespoon oil in a large soup pot over medium heat and add the onion and the remaining 2 teaspoons garlic. Sauté for 5 minutes, stirring frequently.
5. Add the celery and continue to sauté for 10 minutes.
6. Add the chicken broth, beans, tomatoes, and carrots, as well as salt and pepper to taste. Bring the soup to a boil. Cover, decrease the heat, and simmer over low heat for 1 hour.
7. Remove the soup from the heat and let cool for 10 minutes. Working in batches, transfer the soup to a blender or food processor, and puree. Return the blended soup to the pot and cook for 5 minutes over medium heat.
8. Adjust seasonings, if necessary, and serve.

ZUCCHINI SOUP

Makes 4 servings

This soup tastes delicious and is a breeze to make. For a Mexican twist, instead of zucchini, try using chayote. This popular Mexican squash can be found in many large supermarkets.

2 zucchini, cut into chunks

1/2 onion, chopped

1 celery stalk, chopped

1/2 cup shredded Napa cabbage

1 tablespoon minced garlic

1 tablespoon curry powder (optional)

3 cups low-sodium chicken broth

Salt and freshly ground black pepper

Toasted pumpkin seeds, for garnish

1. Combine the zucchini, onion, celery, cabbage, garlic, and curry powder, if using, in a large saucepan. Add the broth and enough water to cover and bring to a boil.
2. Decrease the heat to medium and cook for 20 to 25 minutes, until the vegetables are tender. Remove from the heat and let cool for 10 minutes.
3. Working in batches, transfer the soup to a blender or food processor and process until smooth.
4. Return the blended soup to the pot and cook for 5 more minutes over medium heat. Add salt and pepper to taste.
5. Top each serving with a sprinkle of pumpkin seeds and serve immediately.

Dinners

CHICKEN CURRY WITH VEGGIES ON WHOLE-GRAIN COUSCOUS

Makes 2 servings

This tasty curry goes wonderfully on top of couscous and makes for a filling meal.

2 tablespoons extra virgin olive oil

1/2 onion, chopped

1 tablespoon peeled and chopped ginger

1 garlic clove, minced

1 tablespoon turmeric

1 tablespoon curry powder

1 tablespoon brown sugar

2 5- to 6-ounce skinless, boneless chicken breasts, sliced into 1-inch pieces

1 floret broccoli, chopped

1 small floret of cauliflower, chopped

1 carrot, chopped

1 cup whole-grain couscous, prepared according to instructions on the box

1. Combine the oil, onion, ginger, garlic, turmeric, curry powder, and brown sugar in a large skillet and cook over medium heat until onions turn clear and smell sweet, about 5 minutes.
2. Add the sliced chicken breasts and cook until the meat is done, about 5–7 minutes..
3. Add 1 cup of water along with the broccoli, cauliflower, and carrot. Cook for about 15 minutes, or until the vegetables are tender. Add water as needed to maintain a saucy consistency.
4. Serve over hot, freshly cooked couscous.

CHICKEN ENCHILADAS WITH TOMATO-CILANTRO SAUCE & BLACK BEAN PUREE

Makes 2 servings

Using your blender and a saucepan, you can prepare this impressive traditional dish in very little time. The green tomatoes in the sauce give it a flavor that is totally unique.

SAUCE

6 red or green tomatoes, cut into quarters

2 garlic cloves, chopped

1 serrano or jalapeño chile (optional)

Small handful of fresh cilantro leaves, chopped roughly

1/2 onion, chopped

Salt

ENCHILADAS

1 1-pound bunch fresh spinach, tough stems removed, washed and chopped

2 5- to 6-ounce chicken breasts, boiled, cooled, and then shredded (page 197)

6 stone-ground corn tortillas (make sure they are not flour-based)

Basic Black Beans (page 265) heated and pureed in blender or food processor

1. To make the sauce, fill a medium saucepan one-third full with water and add the tomatoes, half the garlic, and the chile, if using. Bring to a boil, then decrease the heat, and cook on low for about 12 minutes, or until the tomatoes are soft.
2. Transfer about half of the tomatoes and cooking liquid to a blender and add the cilantro, the remaining garlic, and onion. Blend until smooth.
3. Add the remaining tomatoes and cooking liquid and blend on low or pulse for about 1 minute or less to leave some chunky

bits intact. Return to the pan and simmer on low for another 15 minutes, adding salt as needed.

4. To make the enchiladas, place the spinach in a pan and add just enough water to cover. Bring to boil to cook partially and remove immediately with a slotted spoon, or drain.

5. Toss the shredded chicken with the spinach in a mixing bowl.

6. Dip the corn tortillas, one by one, into the sauce and place them on two serving plates. Add 2 tablespoons of the chicken-spinach mixture to each, fold over, and cover with 2 tablespoons of the warm sauce.

7. Serve immediately with a puree of black beans on the side, using additional sauce as needed.

CHICKEN FAJITAS WITH BLACK BEANS, GUACAMOLE, & SALSA MEXICANA

Makes 2 servings

Another traditional Mexican favorite prepared with a healthy BBC twist. Fajitas are a great thing to order when dining out as well—just skip the tortillas and enjoy the healthy filling instead.

1 tablespoon extra virgin olive oil

1/2 green bell pepper, thinly sliced

1/2 onion, sliced

2 5- to 6-ounce skinless, boneless chicken breast halves, cut into
   11/2-inch pieces

Salt and freshly black ground pepper

Basic Black Beans, heated (page 265)

Guacamole (page 266)

Salsa Mexicana (page 267)

1. Heat a nonstick skillet over medium heat. Add the oil, bell pepper, and onion and cook until the onion is clear, about 5 minutes.

2. Add the chicken and stir for another 5 minutes, or until the chicken is cooked through.
3. Remove the pan from the heat and season with salt and pepper to taste. Serve with the black beans, guacamole, and salsa.

CHICKEN STIR-FRY OVER CHOPPED NAPA CABBAGE
Makes 2 servings

Napa cabbage makes this basic stir-fry rich in both flavor and texture and delivers a healthy dose of fiber to fill you up.

1 tablespoon extra virgin olive oil

1 tablespoon toasted sesame oil

1/2 onion, chopped

1 tablespoon peeled, minced ginger

1 clove garlic, minced

1 small head broccoli, cut into spears

8 white button mushrooms, chopped

1 stalk celery, chopped

1 tablespoon low-sodium soy sauce

1/2 cup low-sodium chicken broth

2 5- to 6-ounce boneless, skinless chicken breast halves, sliced

1/2 head Napa cabbage, shredded

1. Heat the olive and sesame oils in a large skillet. Add the onion, ginger, and garlic and sauté over medium heat until the onion turns clear and smells sweet, about 5 minutes.
2. Add the broccoli, mushrooms, celery, soy sauce, and chicken broth and sauté for 2 to 3 minutes.
3. Add the sliced chicken breasts and sauté until the meat is done, about 5–7 minutes.
4. Divide the cabbage between two plates and serve topped with the stir-fry.

FISH KEBABS WITH ZUCCHINI, MUSHROOMS, & CHERRY TOMATOES

Makes 2 servings

The secret to this recipe is to precook the vegetables (except the tomatoes) so that they're done when the fish is cooked. You will need two long or several short skewers to make the kebabs.

MARINADE

1 garlic clove, finely minced

Small handful of cilantro leaves, minced

1/4 cup fresh lemon juice

1 tablespoon extra virgin olive oil

1 tablespoon low-sodium soy sauce (optional)

Salt and freshly ground black pepper

2 5- to 6-ounce white fish fillets, cut into bite-size chunks

1 tablespoon extra virgin olive oil

1/2 red or green bell pepper, diced

1 zucchini, cut into bite-size chunks

1/2 onion, quartered and separated

8 white button mushrooms

8 cherry tomatoes

1 cup whole-grain couscous, prepared according to instructions on the box

1 lemon, quartered

1. To make the marinade, combine the garlic, cilantro, lemon juice, oil, and soy sauce, if using, in a large shallow bowl and whisk together. Add salt and pepper to taste. Add the fish and let it marinate for 30 minutes to 2 hours, turning once.
2. If you are planning to broil your kebabs, preheat the broiler to 500°.
3. To prepare the vegetables, heat the oil in a large skillet over medium heat. Add the bell pepper, zucchini, onion, and mush-

rooms and sauté for 4 to 5 minutes, until slightly tender but not fully cooked.

4. To assemble, thread a tomato, pepper, zucchini, mushroom, and onion piece onto each skewer. Fold over a piece of fish and thread it on. Repeat until the skewer is full.

5. If you do not have a grill, broil the kebabs on a broiler rack or cookie sheet for 6 to 8 minutes, turning once, until cooked through.

6. Serve the kebabs on top of hot, freshly made couscous, garnished with a wedge of lemon.

Bikini Tip

If you are cooking over a gas or charcoal grill and are using wooden skewers, soak them in water for about 30 minutes first to avoid catching the sticks on fire.

FISH TACOS IN LETTUCE "TORTILLAS" WITH SALSA VERDE
Makes 2 servings

Using romaine lettuce leaves as tortillas puts a BBC twist on traditional fish tacos . . . We promise that you won't miss the carbs! Instead of the Salsa Verde, you can serve the tacos with Salsa Mexicana (page 267).

2 5- to 6-ounce grilled white fish fillets (page 197)
1 head romaine lettuce, washed and dried with leaves separated.
Salsa Verde (page 268)

1. Flake the fish into chunks and place in lettuce leaves.
2. Serve with Salsa Verde.

GRILLED FISH WITH MANGO SALSA
Makes 2 servings

The quintessential Caribbean sauce combines sweet mango with spicy serrano chiles to create an irresistible, flavor-packed topping for fish.

1/3 cup diced mango

1/2 cup diced red or yellow bell pepper

1 tablespoon thinly sliced scallions

1 tablespoon chopped cilantro leaves

1 tablespoon diced serrano chile (optional)

1 1-pound bunch fresh spinach

2 5- to 6-ounce grilled white fish fillets (see page 197)

1 teaspoon sliced almonds

1. To make the salsa, combine the mango, bell pepper, scallions, cilantro, and serrano chile, if using, in a bowl. Mix well.
2. To steam the spinach, place the washed leaves (don't shake off or dry) in a hot pan, then cover and steam over medium heat for 2 minutes.
3. Serve the fish on a bed of the spinach, topped with the salsa and sliced almonds.

GRILLED FISH WITH RADISH, CUCUMBER, & JICAMA SALAD
Makes 2 servings

The crunchy, refreshing salad on top contains a hint of lemon and livens up any type of fish.

2 5- to 6-ounce white fish fillets

Easy Lime Marinade (page 262)

SALAD

6 large red radishes, diced

1 cucumber, peeled, seeded, and chopped

1/4 onion, finely minced

1/4 large jicama, peeled and diced

2 tablespoons fresh lemon juice, or to taste

Salt and freshly ground black pepper

1. Place the fish fillets in the marinade in a shallow Tupperware container or baking dish and let sit for 20 to 60 minutes.
2. To make the salad, combine the radishes, cucumber, onion, and jicama in a bowl. Add the lemon juice and mix well. Season with salt and pepper, and more lemon juice, if needed.
3. If using a broiler, preheat to 500°.
4. Broil or grill the fish for about 5 minutes or until cooked on each side.
5. Serve the salad on top of the fish.

GRILLED GINGER SHRIMP WITH ZUCCHINI
Makes 2 servings

Shrimp cook in just minutes, making this an easy dish to prepare when you're pressed for time. The subtle ginger undertones of this recipe mingle nicely with the garlic and zucchini.

2 tablespoons extra virgin olive oil

1 teaspoon peeled, minced ginger

1 teaspoon minced garlic

10 large shrimp, cleaned, tails on and butterflied

1 large zucchini, julienned

2 tablespoons dry white wine

1. Heat the oil in a large skillet over medium heat. Add the ginger and garlic and sauté for 4 to 5 minutes.
2. Add the shrimp, zucchini, and wine, and cook over medium-high heat, stirring frequently, for 3 to 4 minutes, until the shrimp are opaque.
3. Serve immediately.

STEAMED FISH WITH GINGER SAUCE
SERVED OVER SOBA NOODLES

Makes 2 servings

This scrumptious Asian-style dish will have you seeing fish in a whole new light. Remember to keep an eye on the soba noodles, because they can easily overcook.

GINGER SAUCE

1 thumb-size piece ginger, peeled and minced

1 garlic clove, minced

2 tablespoons dry white wine

2 tablespoons low-sodium soy sauce

1 teaspoon toasted sesame oil

1 teaspoon brown sugar

1 small serrano or jalapeño chile, seeded and chopped (optional)

2 5- to 6-ounce white fish fillets

1/2 12-ounce package soba noodles

2 tablespoons chopped fresh cilantro leaves

1 teaspoon toasted sesame seeds

1 thumb-size piece ginger, julienned

1. To make the sauce, combine the ginger, garlic, wine, soy sauce, sesame oil, brown sugar, 1 tablespoon water, and chile pepper, if using, in a bowl. Then transfer to a warm frying pan and cook over medium heat for 5 minutes.
2. Wrap the fish in parchment paper or aluminum foil and place in a metal or bamboo steamer above a pan filled with enough boiling water to cover bottom. Steam for about 6 minutes or until cooked through.
3. Boil the soba noodles in a large pot of salted boiling water according to package instructions, usually about 6 minutes, being careful not to overcook. Drain and run under cool water. Toss with 2 tablespoons of the sauce, or enough to coat the noodles.
4. Remove the fish from its wrapping and serve it on a bed of

soba noodles, drizzled with sauce. Top with cilantro, toasted sesame seeds, and ginger.

STEAMED FISH WITH TOMATOES, PEPPERS, & ONIONS
Makes 2 servings

A BBC variation on a traditional Veracruz-style dish—delicious and simple.

1 tablespoon extra virgin olive oil
1 large green bell pepper, cut into strips
1 large onion, sliced
1 large tomato, sliced
2 5- to 6-ounce white fish fillets

1. Preheat the oven to 350° F.
2. In a large skillet, heat the oil over medium heat. Add the pepper, onion, and tomato and sauté for 4 to 5 minutes, or until the pepper and onion are soft.
3. Lay each fish fillet on a separate piece of aluminum foil or parchment paper. Divide the cooked vegetables on top of each. Fold the foil around the fish so no steam escapes.
4. Place the packets on a baking sheet and bake for about 15 minutes or until the fish is cooked through.
5. Keep the packets closed until serving time to retain the heat, then carefully open each packet and serve.

VEGETABLE FAJITAS WITH BLACK BEANS, GUACAMOLE, & SALSA MEXICANA
Makes 2 servings

A yummy way to get more vegetables into your diet. You won't miss the meat or the carbs!

1 tablespoon extra virgin olive oil

1/2 onion, sliced

1/2 cup sliced white button mushrooms

1 zucchini, julienned

1/2 green bell pepper, thinly sliced

Salt and freshly ground black pepper

Guacamole (page 266)

Basic Black Beans (page 265)

Salsa Mexicana (page 267)

1. Heat the oil in large skillet over medium heat. Add the onion and sauté until tender, about 4 minutes. Add the mushrooms, zucchini, and bell pepper and continue to cook until the peppers are soft, about 5 minutes. Season with salt and pepper.
2. Remove the vegetables from the skillet and serve on plates with Guacamole and Black Beans. Top with Salsa Mexicana.

Desserts

BAKED APPLE WITH BROWN SUGAR & CINNAMON
Makes 2 servings

This sweet treat makes an impressive dessert for guests—simply multiply the recipe, making one apple per person.

2 whole apples

2 teaspoons fresh lemon juice

4 tablespoons raisins

2 tablespoons brown sugar

2 teaspoons cinnamon

1. Preheat the oven to 350° F. Spray a baking dish with nonstick cooking spray.
2. Remove the cores of the apples but do not cut all the way through them so that the bottoms remain intact. Remove ½ inch of the peel at the top of each apple around the hole.
3. Place the apples in the prepared baking dish and sprinkle with the lemon juice to keep them from turning brown.
4. Fill the centers of the apples with raisins and brown sugar. Sprinkle with cinnamon.
5. Bake for 30 to 40 minutes, until soft. Serve warm.

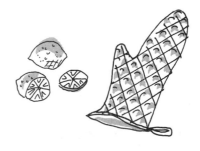

BAKED PEAR WITH BROWN SUGAR & CINNAMON
Makes 2 servings

If pears are not a part of your regular fruit repertoire, this dessert will win you over with its sweet, mild flavor. You want to make sure your pears are ripe; press gently on the flesh with your thumb, and if it gives, the pear is ready to eat. Pears ripen best outside a refrigerator, so if they're firm when you bring them home from the store, leave them in a bowl on your counter to grow soft and juicy.

    2 pears
    2 teaspoons fresh lemon juice
    4 tablespoons raisins
    2 tablespoons brown sugar
    2 teaspoons cinnamon

1. Preheat the oven to 350° F. Spray a baking dish with nonstick cooking spray.
2. Remove the cores of the pears but do not cut all the way through them so that the bottoms remain intact. Remove ½ inch of the peel at the top of each pear around the hole.
3. Place the pears in the prepared baking dish. Sprinkle with the lemon juice.
4. Fill the centers of the pears with the raisins and brown sugar. Sprinkle with cinnamon.
5. Bake for 30 to 40 minutes, until soft. Serve warm.

FRESH BLUEBERRIES WITH MINT
Makes 2 servings

Few people would think to put blueberries and mint together, but this simple dessert hits the spot and is refreshing after any meal.

    2 cups blueberries, washed and chilled
    2 teaspoons minced fresh mint

Combine the blueberries and mint, mix well, divide into 2 portions, and serve immediately.

FRESH MANGO WITH SHREDDED COCONUT
Makes 2 servings

This exotic, very BBC dessert satisfies any sweet tooth!

> 2 mangoes
> 4 ounces shredded unsweetened coconut (or substitute 2 teaspoons grated ginger)

Simply cut up the mangoes as you wish, divide into 2 portions, and sprinkle the coconut on top. Serve immediately.

FRUIT KEBABS
Makes 2 servings

This easy dessert is a great way to use up any leftover fruit you have from other meals. The skewers make for a fun presentation.

> 2 to 3 cups mixed fruit: apples, bananas, pineapples, mangoes, blueberries, pears, or whatever you have lying around
> 2 teaspoons chopped fresh mint or grated ginger (optional)

1. Cut the fruit into bite-sized pieces and thread onto wooden skewers.
2. Sprinkle with fresh mint or a little grated fresh ginger, if desired, and serve.

GRILLED BANANA WITH CARAMEL
Makes 2 servings

This is a another BBC favorite—a sweet treat with a little Mexican flavor. The caramel recalls Mexican dulce de leche. This yummy dessert is guaranteed to satisfy sugar cravings in a healthy, low-calorie way.

2 bananas, peeled
2 tablespoons store-bought caramel sauce

1. Split the banana in half vertically. If the banana is really thick, you can make three vertical slices instead of two.
2. Heat a nonstick skillet over medium-low heat. Add the bananas and cook until a little bit blackened on each side. Do not use oil or butter.
3. Dilute the caramel sauce with 1 tablespoon water. Spoon over the bananas and serve immediately.

HOMEMADE BLUEBERRY SORBET
Makes 2 servings

So easy and satisfying, you will forget that it has almost no calories and fat.

2 cups frozen blueberries
2 cups crushed ice
Sweetener

1. Place the blueberries and ice in a blender and blend on high speed.
2. Add sweetener to taste. Serve immediately.

PINEAPPLE FRAPPÉ
Makes 2 servings

We like to serve these in margarita glasses for fun!

2 cups fresh pineapple chunks
2 cups crushed ice
2 teaspoons chopped fresh mint
Sweetener

1. Place the pineapple, ice, and mint in a blender and blend on high speed, adding sweetener to taste.
2. Serve in margarita glasses with a spoon, or in a bowl.

PINEAPPLE POACHED IN ORANGE JUICE & BROWN SUGAR
Makes 2 servings

The blend of citrus flavors in this recipe balances the sweetness of the brown sugar, and the ginger provides an extra kick. If the ginger flavor doesn't suit you, substitute 1 teaspoon vanilla extract.

1 cup orange juice (fresh is best)
1 tablespoon peeled, minced ginger
2 tablespoons brown sugar
1/2 fresh pineapple, trimmed, cored, and cut into 1/2-inch rings

1. Combine the orange juice, ginger, and brown sugar in a large skillet and cook over low heat for about 15 minutes, until the liquid is reduced by almost half.
2. Add the pineapple and cook for another 5 minutes.
3. Transfer the pineapple to serving bowls, drizzle with the remaining cooking liquid, and serve.

WATERMELON FRAPPÉ

Makes 2 servings

This delicious dessert satisfies the sweet tooth and has almost zero calories!

2 cups cubed watermelon

2 cups crushed ice

Sweetener

1. Place the watermelon and ice in a blender and blend on high speed, adding sweetener to taste.
2. Serve in bowls or margarita glasses.

WHOLE-GRAIN APPLE CRISP

Makes 2 servings

The crunchy texture of the cereal and almonds makes this dessert extremely satisfying.

2 apples, cored and thickly sliced

2 teaspoons fresh lemon juice

2 tablespoons high-fiber cereal

2 tablespoons sliced almonds

4 teaspoons brown sugar

4 teaspoons raisins

1/4 teaspoon cinnamon, plus more as needed

1. Preheat the oven to 350° F.
2. Lay the apples in a shallow baking dish and sprinkle the lemon juice on top.
3. Combine the cereal, almonds, brown sugar, raisins, and cinnamon in a bowl. Spoon over the apples.
4. Bake for 30 minutes, or until the apples are tender.
5. Remove from the heat and sprinkle with more cinnamon, if desired. Serve warm.

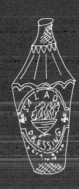

Dressings

All the following recipes serve at least four, so if you are preparing for one or two people, just refrigerate the extra portions for use at a later time. Any of these dressings will make your salads come alive. Always shake well before using.

CITRUS DRESSING
Makes about 1 cup

This tangy delight not only tastes delicious, it's also a great liver cleanser.

1/2 cup fresh lime juice
1/2 cup fresh orange juice
2 tablespoons extra virgin olive oil
Salt and freshly ground black pepper

Combine all the ingredients in a small jar and shake vigorously.

CURRY DRESSING
Makes about 1 cup

Just a dash of this East Indian spice lends ordinary dressing an exotic flavor.

3 tablespoons low-sodium soy sauce
1 tablespoon balsamic vinegar
1/2 cup extra virgin olive oil
1 teaspoon curry powder
2 tablespoons honey

Combine all the ingredients in a blender. Add 1 tablespoon water. Blend on low until smooth. Or, place all the ingredients in a small jar, add 1 tablespoon water, and shake vigorously.

GINGER-SESAME DRESSING
Makes about 1 cup

This yummy dressing is a favorite at Bikini Bootcamp. Try it over salads, fish, and vegetables. You can dilute with water to your liking.

1/2 cup extra virgin olive oil

1/4 cup balsamic vinegar

2 tablespoons low-sodium soy sauce

2 cloves garlic, chopped

2 tablespoons honey or brown sugar

2 tablespoons peeled and minced ginger

1 teaspoon toasted sesame oil

Combine all the ingredients in a blender. Add 2 tablespoons of water. Process until smooth.

MANGO-ORANGE DRESSING
Makes about 1½ cups

A flavorful and fruity addition to any salad.

1/2 mango, chopped

2 tablespoons extra virgin olive oil

1/4 cup orange juice (fresh is best)

1 teaspoon balsamic vinegar

Combine all the ingredients in a blender and blend until smooth.

ORANGE-CILANTRO DRESSING
Makes about ½ cup

The cilantro gives this citrus-based dressing a Mexican twist.

1/4 cup fresh orange juice

2 tablespoons chopped fresh cilantro leaves

1 garlic clove, minced

2 tablespoons extra virgin olive oil

1 tablespoon honey

Combine all the ingredients in a blender and blend on medium speed for about 1 minute. Or place all the ingredients in a small jar with a lid and shake vigorously.

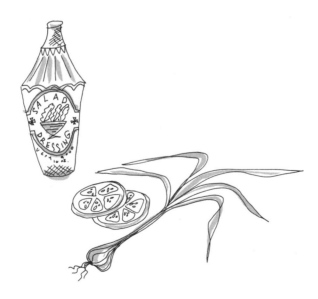

Marinades

These scrumptious marinades turn ordinary fish and chicken into fabulous, yet low-cal, gourmet dishes. The Garlic Cilantro Marinade serves four, so use only as much as you need and refrigerate the rest for later use.

EASY LIME MARINADE
Makes about ½ cup

This one is quick, easy, and perfect for when you're in a rush. It works great with both chicken and fish.

1 garlic clove, minced
Juice of 2 limes
1 tablespoon extra virgin olive oil
1 tablespoon honey
2 tablespoons low-sodium soy sauce
Salt and freshly ground black pepper

Combine all the ingredients and whisk together in a bowl. Simple and delicious!

GARLIC CILANTRO MARINADE
Makes about 1½ cups

A zesty marinade with real Mexican flavor.

1 garlic clove, minced

1 thumb-sized piece of fresh ginger, peeled and minced

1 cup fresh cilantro leaves, minced

1/2 cup fresh lemon juice

3 tablespoons extra virgin olive oil

1 teaspoon low-sodium soy sauce

1/4 cup dry white wine

Pinch of salt and freshly ground black pepper

Whisk together all the ingredients in a bowl.

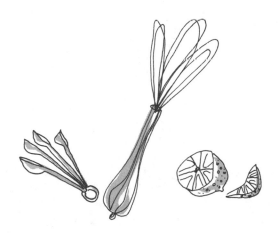

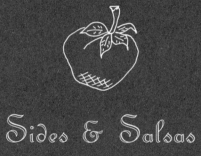

Sides & Salsas

At Bikini Bootcamp we use the following sides and salsas to complement our dishes. These tasty toppings will give your food that extra-special Mexican zip—plus grade-A nutrition—without packing on the pounds. They add real flavor to your food so you'll never feel deprived.

BASIC BLACK BEANS
Makes 2 servings

Black beans are a classic Mexican dish and make for a wonderful side to complement any meal. They are also packed with fiber.

1 cup dried black beans, picked over, rinsed, and soaked overnight

1/2 cup chopped white onion

2 tablespoons extra virgin olive oil

1 teaspoon salt

1. Combine the beans, onion, oil, and 9 cups water in a 3-quart saucepan. Bring to a boil, reduce the heat, and simmer, partially covered, for 1¼ hours, or until the beans are tender.
2. Add the salt and simmer, uncovered, until enough water has evaporated so that liquid reaches just below the level of the beans, about 30 minutes.
3. Serve hot.

Bikini Tip
If you don't have time to cook your beans from scratch, just rinse and drain a 15-ounce can black beans. Sauté the onion in 4 teaspoons olive oil in a small heavy saucepan over low heat, stirring frequently, for 4 to 5 minutes, or until softened. Stir in the beans and 1/2 cup water and simmer for 15 minutes.

GUACAMOLE

Makes 2–4 servings

Whenever you prepare guacamole, always keep the pit in the bowl to prevent it from turning brown too soon.

1 avocado, halved, pitted, and peeled (reserve the pit)
1 fresh serrano chile, seeded and minced (optional)
2 tablespoons fresh lime juice
1 tomato, chopped
Salt and freshly ground black pepper

1. Combine the avocado, chile, if using, lime juice, and tomato in a medium bowl, and mash with a fork until almost smooth.
2. Season to taste with salt and pepper and serve.

HUMMUS

Makes 2–4 servings

Hummus is a great side dish served with any crisp veggies, such as cucumber, carrot, or jicama, or on whole-grain crisps that are fiber-rich, such as Ak-Mak brand crackers. You can buy fresh hummus or make your own, using our delicious recipe that follows. It lasts for at least a week and makes a healthy snack. You can also play with this basic recipe by adding cilantro, jalapeño, or roasted red peppers.

1 (15-ounce) can chickpeas (garbanzo beans), drained
1 teaspoon chopped garlic
Juice of 1 lime
1 tablespoon extra virgin olive oil
Salt

1. Combine the chickpeas, garlic, lime juice, and oil in a blender

or food processor and blend on high speed until smooth. You may need to drizzle in a bit of water if it looks too thick.

2. Season to taste with salt and serve.

SALSA MEXICANA

Makes 4 servings

Salsa brightens any meal and can be used to top hard-boiled eggs, fish, and salads.

4 medium tomatoes, chopped

1/2 large onion, chopped

1/4 cup minced fresh cilantro leaves

2 tablespoons fresh lime juice

1/2 jalapeño or serrano chile, seeded and minced

Salt and freshly ground black pepper

1. Combine the tomatoes, onion, cilantro, lime juice, and chile in a medium bowl and mix well.
2. Season to taste with salt and pepper. Keep chilled.

Bikini Tip
It's best not to keep fresh salsa for more than a day or two, because the tomatoes tend to become acidic.

SALSA VERDE (GREEN AVOCADO SAUCE)
Makes 2–4 servings

An excellent topping for tacos, salads, and vegetables. To use as a marinade or topping for fish, add 2 tablespoons of olive oil. Note that this particular sauce should not be kept for more than one day, and is best used within several hours.

1 avocado, chopped
2 garlic cloves, minced
1 serrano chile, minced (optional)
1/2 onion, chopped
1 small handful fresh cilantro leaves

Combine the avocado, garlic, chile, onion, cilantro, and 4 tablespoons of water in a blender and process until smooth.

SPICY BLACK BEAN DIP
Makes 2–4 servings

This easy condiment is a great way to jazz up healthy snacks like carrot, cucumber, and celery sticks.

1/2 (15-ounce) can black beans, drained and rinsed
1 small jalapeño chile, seeded and diced
1 medium tomato, diced
Salt and freshly ground black pepper

1. Combine all the ingredients in a bowl and mix well.
2. Transfer to a food processor or blender and blend until smooth. Season with salt and pepper.

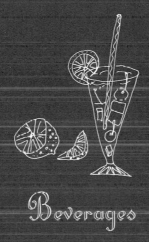

Beverages

At Bikini Bootcamp, we are very proud of our low-cal, absolutely delicious drinks, and our guests are always clamoring for the recipes. Once you taste them, you will never, ever turn to sodas, sugared fruit juices, or even those chemical-laden sports drinks that are all the rage. In all of these recipes, we recommend sweetening with stevia, a natural, noncaloric, and safe sweetener derived from a plant. Stevia is found in most health-food stores. Just keep in mind that stevia is sweeter than sugar, so a little goes a long way!

GINGER LIMEADE
Makes 1 serving

Nothing is more refreshing—or better for cleansing and stimulating your digestion—than a ginger drink, which we serve to our guests as soon as they arrive. You can also serve it with a sprig of fresh mint on the side.

1 cup fresh lime or lemon juice
1 finger-size piece ginger, peeled and finely minced
Sweetener

1. Dilute the fresh lime juice with water to taste and combine with 1 tablespoon of the ginger in a blender.
2. Add sweetener and blend on high for 2 minutes.
3. Adjust the amount of ginger and sweetener to taste and serve.

Bikini Tip

If you want a change from ginger, you can add a small handful of washed and crushed mint leaves instead. You can also make this drink into a slushy by adding ice and blending.

HIBISCUS TEA
Serves 4

A BBC favorite! Our guests are always dying to know what this unusual and tasty beverage is and how we make it. Hibiscus tea is actually a typ-

ical Mexican beverage that is said to have blood-cleansing properties. You can find hibiscus leaves in health-food, Mexican, and gourmet-food stores.

1 small handful hibiscus leaves

Sweetener

1. Boil the hibiscus leaves in 4 cups water for 3 minutes on high, then decrease the heat and let the tea simmer for another minute.
2. Turn off the heat completely and let the tea steep. The longer it steeps, the stronger it will be. You can also dilute with more water if you prefer.
3. Add sweetener to taste and serve hot.

Bikini Tip

Chill your Hibiscus Tea during the summertime for a supreme cool-down drink!

MINT TEA
Serves 2

The classic refresher, mint tea is a delicious drink that also soothes a troubled tummy. It can be served hot or chilled.

1 small handful fresh mint leaves

Sweetener

1. Boil the fresh mint leaves in 2 cups water for 3 minutes on high, then decrease the heat, and let the tea simmer for another minute.
2. Turn off the heat completely and let the tea steep. Dilute with water to your liking.
3. Add sweetener, such as stevia, to taste, and serve hot or chilled.

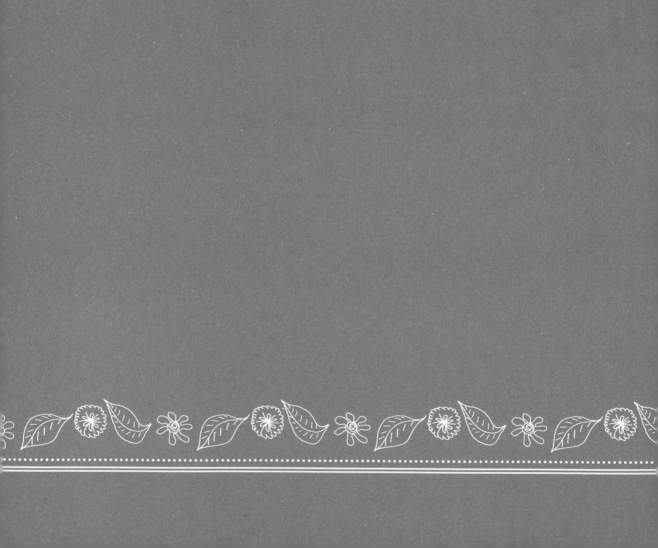

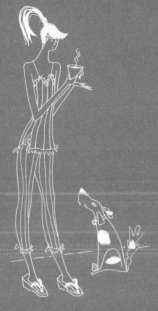

PART IV

Living the Lifestyle

There is no shortage of good days. It is good lives that are hard to come by.
—*Annie Dillard*

Congratulations—you did it! The past fourteen days have been challenging and intense, but we hope that by now you're feeling the pleasures of being in your slimmer, shapelier bikini body. Your pants are fitting looser, your energy has skyrocketed, and you likely have muscles you've never had before. We bet you're even standing taller on account of your yoga workouts and newly toned core. If you're like most of our campers, you're feeling pretty good about yourself—and you should! After all your hard work, you're ready to hit the beach.

If, however, you're not quite as toned as you'd like, or still have more pounds to lose, don't worry. The changes you see will obviously vary depending on your starting weight and fitness level. If you started the program a size twelve, you can't expect to be a size two in just two weeks, no matter how hard you've been working out. What you can expect is to see the beginnings of bigger changes already taking place—you've given your body a jump-start in terms of losing weight, and if you continue to follow the Bikini Bootcamp meal plans and exercise routines laid out in Part II, the pounds will continue to disappear. Remember, our program is designed to be a lifestyle that you embrace long after these fourteen days are up, whether you've reached your optimum shape or have more work to do. In this section, we'll tell you how to either maintain your new-found figure all year round, or keep making progress to reach your fitness and weight-loss goals.

Keep It Coming Off

If you've had a good start on the fourteen-day plan but have not yet reached your ideal weight, that's okay—you can continue to melt away the pounds simply by repeating the two-week plan in Part II. Unlike fad diets, our meal plan is balanced in proteins, carbs, healthy fats, and everything else you need to keep your body working properly, so remaining on it over time won't undermine your health in any way. You can safely repeat the two weeks as many times as it takes to achieve your desired shape; on average, you can expect to lose two to three pounds a week, and with results like that you'll be motivated to stay the course.

If you'd like a little more variety in your meals, or are simply too busy to whip up our recipes from scratch every day, check out the BBC Eating

Plan for Girls on the Go on page 284. This simplified plan offers suggestions for what to eat when you're in a rush or away from your own kitchen to ensure that you're keeping the calorie count down and getting the same amounts of protein, fiber, and healthy fats that you would on a regular BBC plan. These creative options make it easy to stick with the program and keep the pounds coming off.

You should also continue with the regular workout regimen as outlined in Parts I and II: circuit training, yoga, and walking every day; core strengthening three times a week. If you want, you can opt for an hour-long yoga class twice a week rather than 15 minutes on your own every day. Finding a supportive yoga teacher and community can be another terrific way to bolster your efforts as you continue to transform your shape. With each passing week, your body will become noticeably firmer and more toned.

We also recommend that you keep up with your meditations and journal writing so you can stay focused on getting the results you want. And don't forget to reward yourself along the way for a job well done! Whether you follow our at-home recipes for pampering or treat yourself to massages, facials, and mani-pedis at a spa, always lavish your body with care and gratitude for everything it has given you, and for carrying you into this new chapter of your life.

Maintaining Your Bikini Body

If the two-week plan has done the job, and you're feeling energized and confident and ready to go—fantastic! But you don't want to let all your hard work go to waste, or slip back into bad habits. We want you to continue to make smart choices about how you fuel your body and the amount of exercise you get throughout the day. We've been living the BBC lifestyle for years and can attest firsthand that it is both sustainable and pleasurable! So whether you're a permanent beach bunny, a career girl, or a mother of five, our maintenance plan will keep you slim, sexy, bikini-ready, and above all *healthy* for years to come.

How Often Should You Work Out?
Let's be honest—you can't slip back into old negative habits on Day 15 and expect to keep your bikini shape. So even though you no longer have

to exercise every single day, you want to be sure to continue with your workouts in order to keep your metabolism revved and your muscles toned. Even a week or two of slacking off can slow your metabolism and lead to diminished muscle mass. So follow our maintenance workout regimen to ensure that the numbers on the scale don't start creeping up—and that you retain your BBC glow:

Circuit Training: 3 times a week. When you're pressed for time, follow our special "At the Office or On the Road" circuit training routine on page 277.

Core Strengthening: 2 times a week.

Yoga: A least 15 minutes of Sun Salutations 3 times a week *or* take 2 weekly yoga classes at a local studio.

Walking: A minimum of 30 minutes (one hour is ideal) at a brisk pace, 3 times a week.

Remember to intersperse your workouts with other activities you enjoy that also give you plenty of exercise: dance classes, bike rides, hiking, or even rock climbing or surfing. As you continue to build strength and endurance, you'll find a door opening to all sorts of fun physical activities you've never done before, and challenging your body in new ways will become a pleasure. Try to do something different at least twice a month, and involve your friends and family when you can.

Here are a few other things to keep in mind:

• Adjust the level of your hand weights as you get stronger, working up to eight pounds. You don't need more weight than that to get results.
• On your walks, try some of our suggestions from Chapter 4 as you become more advanced. Walk with a weighted vest to up the caloric burn, tackle hilly terrain, or do some basic interval training: alternate 10 minutes of walking with 5 minutes of running, 2 minutes of lunges, jumping rope, or anything else that suits your fancy and keeps your heart rate up.
• With your Sun Salutations, move up through the different levels of routines in Chapter 3 and increase the number and speed of the flows as you are able.

Bikini Tip ···

Try pairing your walking and circuit training for an extended circuit from time to time!

···

Circuit Training:
At the Office or On the Road

On those days when you can't spare a moment from work, squeeze in some time for the following lunch-hour routine in your office or cubicle. The only equipment you need is your desk and two full one-liter water bottles. As with our previous circuit training routines, you'll alternate 1 minute of each of the strength moves with 2 minutes of cardio—either marching or jogging in place, depending upon how hard you want to work.

CARDIO: 2 MINUTES. March or jog in place (if you are want to avoid working up too much of a sweat or if you have bad knees, stick to marching in place).

PLIÉ SQUATS: 1 MINUTE (targets inner thighs and glutes)

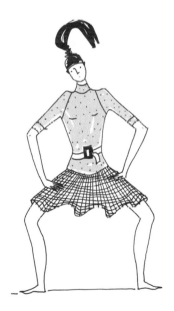

- Stand with your feet apart, slightly wider than your hips, with your toes pointing outward.
- Bend your knees and lower yourself, keeping your back straight and your abs slightly contracted.
- Straighten your knees and return to the starting position. Repeat for 1 minute.

Advanced: Hold a large, full water bottle with both hands, and raise the bottle to chest level by bending your elbows while squatting down.

TRICEP DIPS: 1 MINUTE (targets triceps and core muscles)

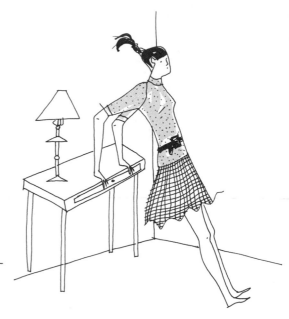

- Stand with your back to your desk, hands at your sides, palms facing down and positioned directly beneath your shoulders. Grip the edge of the desk with your fingertips. Your legs are extended out straight, so that your heels are on the floor, toes are pointing up, and there is about 3 feet of space between your toes and the edge of the desk.
- Bend your elbows and lower yourself down so your hips dip below the desktop, keeping your back close to the edge.
- Straighten your arms and return to the starting position. Remember, the lift is done with your arm muscles (triceps), not your legs. Repeat for 1 minute.

KNEE LIFTS: 1 MINUTE (targets abs and shoulders)

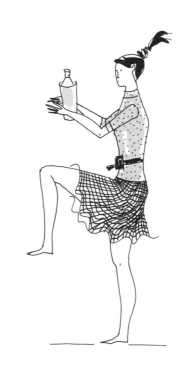

- Stand with your feet hip-width apart, holding a full water bottle with both hands.
- Extend your arms overhead, keeping a slight bend in your elbows.
- Now lift your left knee as you lower your arms so the bottle and your knee meet just above hip-height.
- Lower your left knee, and raise your arms back overhead.
- Repeat on your right side, and keep alternating legs for 1 minute.

CARDIO: 2 MINUTES. March or jog in place.

REVERSE LUNGES: 1 MINUTE

(target glutes and hamstrings)

- Stand with your back about 1 1/2 feet from a wall.
- Your feet are planted flat on the ground. Step back with your left foot so your heel touches the wall.
- Bend both your knees, leaning slightly forward as your hips shift back toward the wall, as if you were in the process of sitting down. Do not actually touch the wall with your back or hips.
- Come up to the standing position. Repeat for 30 seconds.
- Switch sides.

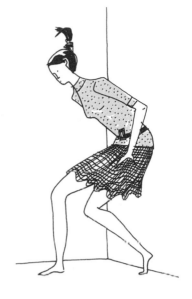

CRISS-CROSS ARMS: 1 MINUTE

(targets shoulders and lats)

- Stand with your feet hip-width apart, your knees slightly bent.
- Holding a full water bottle in each hand, raise your arms straight out in front of your chest, elbows slightly bent.
- Now, criss-cross your arms, keeping your fists close to each other and your wrists level, rather than bent up or down. Lower only when it's time to move on to the next exercise.

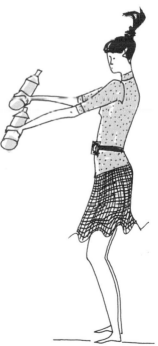

SIDE EXTENSIONS: 1 MINUTE (targets core, shoulders, and abdominal obliques)

- Stand with your feet hip-width apart, knees slightly bent.
- Hold a full water bottle with both hands.
- Extend your arms and the bottle overhead, keeping your elbows slightly bent.
- Now lean to the right, tilting your body and the bottle slightly forward, as far as you can.
- Return to the center starting position and repeat on the left. Repeat, alternating sides, for 1 minute.

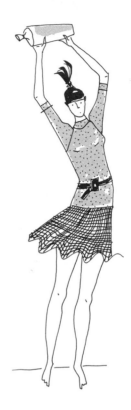

CARDIO: 2 MINUTES. March or jog in place.

WALL SITS: 1 MINUTE (targets hamstrings and glutes)

- Stand with your legs hip-width apart and lean back against a wall.
- Sit down as if you were in an imaginary chair. Make sure your knees are in line with your hips, your knees directly over your ankles and hip-width apart. Hold for 1 minute.

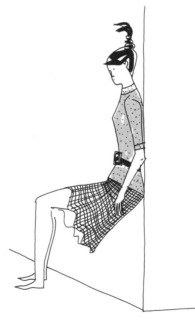

DESK PUSH-UPS: 1 MINUTE (targets chest, shoulders, and biceps)

- Stand about 3 feet away from your desk and place your hands on its edge, shoulder-width apart.
- Extend your legs straight behind you, hip-width apart, with the balls of your feet pressed down on the floor. Your torso should be straight but at a slight angle toward the desk.
- Now bend your elbows, keeping them close to your ribs, and lower your chest toward the desk, keeping your core engaged and your back straight by pulling your navel toward your spine throughout the exercise.
- Return to the start position and repeat.

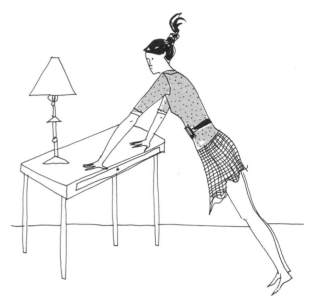

KNEE LIFTS: 1 MINUTE (targets abs and shoulders)

- Stand with your feet hip width apart, holding a full water bottle with both hands.
- Extend your arms overhead, keeping a slight bend in your elbows.
- Now lift your right knee as you lower your arms so the bottle and your knee meet just above hip-height.
- Lower your right knee, and raise your arms back overhead.
- Repeat on your left side and keep alternating legs for 3 minutes.

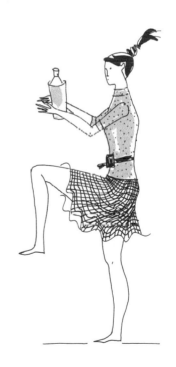

CARDIO: 2 MINUTES. March or jog in place.

REPEAT the entire circuit, and there you go—a full circuit-training routine that can be done wherever you are.

Other Office Exercises ....

- Skip the elevator and take the stairs.
- Stand up and do a few squats or lunges while you are on the phone. Every little bit helps!
- Use your lunch hour for a brisk walk (keep a pair of sneakers stashed in a desk drawer).
- Take the longer, scenic route to the lunchroom or the copy machine, or take the stairs to use the bathroom on a higher floor.

....

What Should You Eat?

Now that you've completed the fourteen-day jump-start, you can be a bit more flexible in your eating habits. However, in order to maintain your newfound bikini shape, you'll want to stay true to the Bikini Bootcamp philosophy and continue "Living the Lifestyle" even after these first two weeks are done:

- Try not to eat foods that are more than one step away from their source by the time they reach your plate. Avoid processed and refined foods, and buy organic produce, chicken, and eggs whenever possible.
- Have some protein at every meal. Bear in mind that protein is not found only in eggs, beans, and meats—it is also found in yogurt, low-fat milk, flax seed, nuts, soy, and some grains. You should aim for at least one serving of fish or chicken every day, and make sure that your other meals contain protein as well, even if it's only in the form of a handful of almonds or a few spoonfuls of yogurt over fruit.
- Keep your diet high in fiber. Try to opt for a salad at lunch; eat a wide variety of fruits and veggies, approximately six to eight servings (or cups) a day; and make sure that any grains you eat contain at least 4 grams of fiber per serving.
- Have a healthy snack in the afternoon to keep your metabolism supercharged. Counteract that afternoon chocolate craving with nuts, fruits, and other favorites from our BBC snack list on page 194.

As we've said, many of our campers return home to find themselves adopting our way of eating automatically—they feel so good and so healthy that their bodies just don't want to stop! You can continue to enjoy your favorite recipes from our cookbook section and experiment with others that make use of similar ingredients and are low-fat, low-cal, and high-fiber in nutritional content. There are countless variations to be made with our staple BBC foods listed on pages 186–193, so have fun whipping up your own creative dishes. Before long, you'll have an intuitive sense of which foods serve your body best—and lose your taste for the ones that don't.

Here are some of the most frequently asked questions from BBC grads about adapting the meal plan to their lifestyle:

IS IT EVER OKAY TO HAVE REAL DESSERTS—CAKES, COOKIES, CHOCOLATE—OR REFINED SUGAR?

If you're eating healthy most of the time and your weight is stable, an occasional treat won't sabotage your success. The key is moderation, so watch your portion size and mind that you don't indulge too often. Remember, it doesn't take much to satisfy your sweet tooth—a single square of high-quality, dark chocolate (which has antioxidant properties, unlike milk chocolate) can give you the taste sensation you crave as easily as a Hostess Twinkie—and with far fewer calories. If you're out to dinner with friends, splitting dessert is an easy way to make sure that you don't overindulge. Or, simply have a bite of someone else's and sip a mint tea instead.

IS IT EVER OKAY TO HAVE RED MEAT?

Yes, red meat provides iron and quality protein; however, it also contains saturated fats, which have been linked to heart disease and clogged arteries. Recent studies also suggest a link between high consumption of red meat and certain types of cancers. You should limit red meat to twice a week, and then only in a fist-sized portion. Try to eat lean, organic meat, which means that the animal was not given antibiotics or hormones, and in the case of beef, opt for grass-fed whenever possible, which means that the animal was allowed to graze freely.

WHAT ABOUT BREADS, PASTA, AND OTHER CARBS?

Again, the key is moderation in both frequency and portion size. Carbs are not the enemy—after all, as we've seen, they're a valuable source of energy and nutrients. The key is to opt for those with a high fiber count. Today, healthier versions of classic carbs are easily found in supermarkets—whole-wheat pasta for example, for when you're craving Italian, or organic, multigrain breads that actually taste great. When buying packaged foods—cereals, crackers, breads—always remember to look for brands that contain at least 4 grams of fiber per serving.

The BBC Eating Plan for Girls on the Go

If you're one of those women who's constantly on the go and rarely at home long enough to sleep, let alone shop for food and prepare breakfast, lunch, and dinner from scratch, there are still ways to make the Bikini Bootcamp program work for you. We call this our section for Girls on the Go, so if you aren't able to follow the meal plan letter by letter, or if you eat out a lot during the week, you can use the suggestions listed here to stay on the BBC track. They can be used any time you're in a pinch during the initial two-week program, and also after the first two weeks are up, to maintain your hard-earned bikini figure.

BREAKFAST CHOICES:

Fruit Smoothie: Smoothies are a great, easy breakfast when you're in a rush, and if you add some flax seed, you'll get your protein boost as well. Experiment with different fruits using the recipes in the cookbook section.
Eggs: Two scrambled, poached, or hard-boiled eggs with fruit on the side.
Yogurt: 1 cup low-fat yogurt with 1/2 cup fruit or a tablespoon of high-fiber cereal.

LUNCH CHOICES:

Soup: Opt for a vegetable- or chicken-broth base, never cream. If you're eating soup as your main course, try to include some protein as well: beans, chicken, fish, or shrimp.
Turkey sandwich on multigrain, high-fiber bread (if in doubt about whether the bread is high-fiber, ask to see the package): With mustard (never mayo), lettuce, tomato, and any other veggies that are available.
Turkey or veggie burger on a bed of lettuce and tomatoes
Green salad with chicken or fish, dressing on the side: Load up on the dark

leafy greens like spinach, and opt for olive oil and vinegar rather than a creamy dressing; 1 tablespoon is usually sufficient.

Grilled chicken, black beans, and fresh salsa: You can ask any restaurant to hold the tortilla.

One 6-ounce can of white-meat tuna packed in water with vegetables or salad on the side.

SNACK CHOICES:

Fresh fruit: 1 piece, or 1 cup of smaller fruits like grapes and berries.

DINNER CHOICES:

6 ounces of grilled, poached, or steamed chicken or fish, with vegetables and brown rice or any fiber-rich grain on the side: When ordering meat, be sure to request that they use a minimal amount of oil in the preparation. If the dish includes a sauce, ask that it be left off as the base of most sauces is butter or hidden oil. If possible, ask them to prepare your fish with lemon or lime and salt and pepper.

Green salads with lean protein such as beans, fish, or chicken, dressing on the side: Salad with any kind of vegetables makes a perfect meal; just be sure that it doesn't include cheese or anything fried or sautéed, such as bacon or croutons. You can always ask the chef to hold any unhealthy ingredients like bacon.

Chicken Paillard: Grilled chicken breast with arugula and tomatoes on top.

Chinese chicken salad: Order it without the crispy wontons, and with the dressing on the side so you can control the amount you use.

Grilled chicken fajitas with black beans and salsa: Ask for corn tortillas, which are lower in calories and higher in fiber than flour ones. And skip the sour cream!

Taco salad with grilled chicken, fish, or black beans, lettuce and salsa: Order without the taco shell, sour cream, and cheese.

Sashimi with low-sodium soy sauce, edamame, and a green salad: Sashimi is sushi but without the rice—a perfect low-cal source of protein. Order a side of edamame and a salad for additional protein and fiber.

DESSERT CHOICES:

Fresh fruit: 1 piece, or 1 cup of smaller fruits like grapes and berries.

Herbal tea: Herbal teas such as mint, chamomile, lemon, ginger, and cinnamon make for a nice end to a meal if you want to avoid the calories altogether.

Remember, the Bikini Bootcamp way of eating is designed to be manageable for the long haul. As we said in Chapter 5, the word "failure" does not exist in the BBC vocabulary. So if you feel like you've let your eating or exercise habits slip—whether around the holidays or on a luxurious trip with lots of meals at fabulous restaurants—simply "begin again."

What About Journaling and Meditation?

As you wind down the intensive BBC plan and your busy life returns to normal, you might find yourself tempted to skip these extra activities. And while you certainly don't need to do them every day, we encourage you to continue to make them a part of your life. Why? Because in addition to their role in changing your eating and fitness habits, they provide easy and simple ways to nurture your spirit and escape from the chaos of everyday life. We can't all pack our bags and head to the beaches of Tulum whenever we need a break, but journaling and meditation can help you create a sense of serenity, perspective, and clarity wherever you are.

A Final Word

Before we leave you, we'd like to tell you about the "Closing Ceremony" that we have for our guests on their final night of Bikini Bootcamp. We sit with our campers and dogs in a candlelit circle on the beach, and we ask everyone in turn to think of a word or phrase—kind of like a mantra—that they can take home with them in order to remain connected to their Bikini Bootcamp experience. Some of the words that our guests share include "balance," "strength," "motivation," and "challenge," and some of the phrases we hear include "I will not worry about my job," "I will keep making healthy choices," and "I will remember what it felt like to exercise and love it." We also hear a slew of other happy revelations as our campers rave: "I've never felt this good in my life," "My body's never felt this way," and "I've never looked so good!"

What's your word or phrase? Pick something that reminds you of everything you've accomplished over the past two weeks, and of how great you look and feel in your new bikini body. Keep this word or phrase with you in the weeks and months that follow—even when the winter weather sets in—to ensure that you continue exercising and nourishing your body and remain fit, strong, healthy, and radiant, always.

We invite you to come see us at Amansala in Mexico to share your experience with us firsthand, and to meet other Bikini Bootcampers who've been enjoying the program just like you. Our guests make up our extended family and are an intricate part of what makes BBC so special. In the meantime, we wish you good health, good eating, and tremendous success in every aspect of your life. You've done great work. See you on the beach!

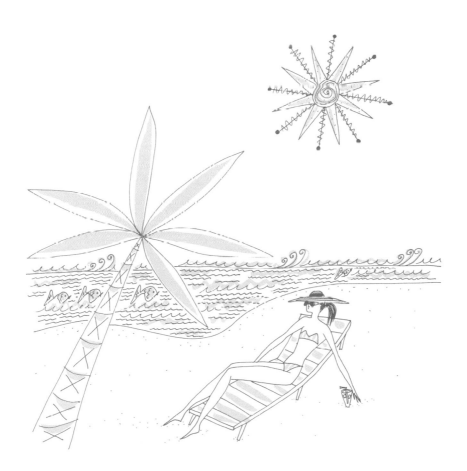

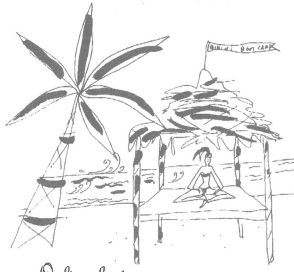

Bikini Bootcamp Online

LOSE WEIGHT FASTER

Achieve your ultimate beach body while having fun! That's what the Bikini Bootcamp is all about. And to make it easier, we've just launched the Bikini Bootcamp Online program, which can enhance your results and customize your experience.

Gain access to fun and interactive online tools that will track your progress and record your results; meet an online community that will offer daily support and diet tips; and receive advice and info on new topics from the authors, Erica and Melissa.

Bikini Tip...

Studies show that people who participate in online weight-loss programs — such as the Bikini Bootcamp Online — have more success than those who go it alone. What are you waiting for?

Online features

* Daily Meal Planner
* Custom Fitness Plan
* 100s of New Recipes
* Community Support
* Q&As with the Authors

Online benefits

* Lose Weight
* Feel Healthier
* Tone Your Body
* Have Fun
* Get Your Beach Body!

Get a Free Bikini Makeover...

As a thank-you for purchasing the book, we're giving you a special online Bikini Makeover. Go ahead — reach your goals!

www.bikinibootcamp.com/book

Visit the above Web site to get a special offer. Offer expires December 31, 2008.

Acknowledgments

It takes a village to raise a child, and Bikini Bootcamp was our first child. We want to extend our gratitude to the BBC staff and to all of the guests who have visited with us over the years.

We would also like to thank Ann Campbell, our fabulous editor at Broadway Books, for being a true Bikini Bootcamp believer; Elena Oumano for her patience in assisting us with writing this book; Jennifer Joel, our dedicated agent at ICM; and all the Broadway Books crew, especially Julia Coblentz, Tammy Blake, and Laura Lee Mattingly, who helped make this dream a reality.

From Erica.
I would like to extend gratitude to my parents, Angela and Eric, for their unwavering support and love. Thank you for giving me wings. Thanks also to my incredibly supportive friends in San Francisco and New York City (you all know who you are); to Better-Than-Bond, for the laughter and lessons; and to the yoga teachers and trainers who have inspired me along the way (especially Karin in San Francisco). I would also like to thank Melissa, for being a great friend and business partner . . . What a magical adventure!

About the Authors

Melissa Perlman studied Tibetan Buddhism in Asia for more than six years and owned a restaurant in Tokyo that served healthy California cuisine. **Erica Gragg** is a former public relations executive and certified yoga and fitness instructor. Friends for eight years, in 2002 Melissa and Erica founded the Amansala Eco-Chic Resort and Bikini Bootcamp, which now boasts more than 3,000 guests a year.